DENTAL HYGIENE PROCESS
DIAGNOSIS AND CARE PLANNING

DENTAL HYGIENE PROCESS:
DIAGNOSIS AND CARE PLANNING

Laura Mueller-Joseph, BSDH, MS
Assistant Professor
State University of New York at Farmingdale
Department of Dental Hygiene

Marie Petersen, RDH, MS
Associate Professor
State University of New York at Farmingdale
Department of Dental Hygiene

Delmar Publishers ™

I(T)P° An International Thomson Publishing Company

Albany • Bonn • Boston • Cincinnati • Detroit • London • Madrid • Melbourne
Mexico City • New York • Pacific Grove • Paris • San Francisco • Singapore • Tokyo
Toronto • Washington

NOTICE TO THE READER

Publisher does not warrant or guarantee any of the products described herein or perform any independent analysis in connection with any of the product information contained herein. Publisher does not assume, and expressly disclaims, any obligation to obtain and include information other than that provided to it by the manufacturer.

The reader is expressly warned to consider and adopt all safety precautions that might be indicated by the activities described herein and to avoid all potential hazards. By following the instructions contained herein, the reader willingly assumes all risks in connection with such instructions.

The publisher makes no representations or warranties of any kind, including but not limited to, the warranties of fitness for particular purpose or merchantability, nor are any such representations implied with respect to the material set forth herein, and the publisher takes no responsibility with respect to such material. The publisher shall not be liable for any special, consequential or exemplary damages resulting, in whole or in part, from the readers' use of, or reliance upon, this material.

Cover: Douglas Hyldelund

Delmar Staff
Acquisitions Editor: Kimberly Davies
Assistant Editor: Debra Flis
Project Editor: Melissa Conan
Production Coordinator: Mary Ellen Black
Editorial Assistant: Donna Leto
Production Services: Publishers' Design and Production Services, Inc.

COPYRIGHT © 1995
By Delmar Publishers
A division of International Thomson Publishing Inc.
The ITP logo is a trademark under license
Printed in the United States of America

For more information, contact:

Delmar Publishers
3 Columbia Circle, Box 15015
Albany, NY 12212-5015

International Thomson Publishing Europe
Berkshire House 168-173
High Holborn
London WC1V7AA
England

Thomas Nelson Australia
102 Dodds Street
South Melbourne, 3205
Victoria, Australia

Nelson Canada
1120 Birchmount Road
Scarborough, Ontario
Canada M1K 5G4

International Thomson Editores
Campos Eliseos 385, Piso 7
Col Polanco
11560 Mexico D F Mexico

International Thomson Publishing GmbH
Königswinterer Strasse 418
53227 Bonn
Germany

International Thomson Publishing Asia
221 Henderson Road
#05-10 Henderson Building
Singapore 0315

International Thomson Publishing—Japan
Hirakawacho Building, 3F
2-2-1 Hirakawacho
Chiyoda-ku, Tokyo 102
Japan

2 3 4 5 6 7 8 9 10 XXX 01 00 99 98 97 96 95

Library of Congress Cataloging-in-Publication Data

Mueller-Joseph, Laura,
    Dental hygiene process: diagnosis and care planning / by Laura Mueller-Joseph, Marie
Petersen.
        p.   cm.
    Includes bibliographical references and index.
    ISBN 0-8273-5678-1
    1. Dental hygiene. I. Petersen, Marie. II. Title.
    [DNLM: 1. Dental Care. 2. Patient Care Planning. 3. Dental Hygienists. WU 29
M947d 1995]
    617.6'01'68—dc20   94-32214
                                                                     CIP

TO

My husband,
David, for his love,
support, and encouragement.

My parents,
Kurt and Lillian Mueller, for
their guidance and wisdom.

My sister,
Karen Mueller, who has always
been there during the
laughter and the tears.

– LMJ –

My husband,
Herb, whose support and
love surround me.

The generations of my
family who are my foundation.

All the students
who have taught me so well.

– MEP –

Irene Woodall
whose inspiration and
insight has helped direct the
dental hygiene profession to the future.

CONTENTS

PREFACE

This text is written for the dental hygiene student in the second year of clinical education, although a portion of it may be introduced in the first year. It would also be extremely useful for a hygienist returning to the profession after a period of retirement, or a practicing hygienist who wants to improve upon his or her diagnostic and treatment planning skills. The text uses the conceptual framework of the process of dental hygiene care, which moves from assessment, diagnosis, planning, and implementation to evaluation. It is meant to be used as a companion text to any of those that cover the fundamentals of dental hygiene practice.

The text was written by two educators who have felt through their own experience and conversations with colleagues that in the majority of educational settings students must learn a large volume of diverse material in the biomedical and dental sciences, psychology, and communication. This is in addition to learning clinical skills, techniques, and protocols of treatment in a very intense manner. Students may feel overwhelmed by the volume of information, and faculty complain that the student has a hard time "putting it all together." This text is written to help the student or the practicing hygienist use clinical and scientific theory in a manner dedicated to the identification of conditions relevant to the hygienist's unique practice.

The text chapters follow the five phases of the dental hygiene process of care. An introductory chapter defines the conceptual framework of the process. Chapter 2 reviews assessment by categorizing the types of data that may be collected. The third chapter, Dental Hygiene Diagnosis, may be new to many. Dental hygienists have historically been taught in certain instances that the term "diagnosis" was not to be used and was the purview of the dentist. However, dental hygiene practice standards in place for more than a decade have clearly identified diagnoses of conditions that the dental hygienist is competent to treat. The chapter further defines the difference between the dental and dental hygiene diagnoses and gives many examples. Planning for care is divided into two chapters. The fourth chapter describes care planning using an epidemiological approach that categorizes disease and helps to determine the type of intervention. This chapter also reviews three models of health behavior and their clinical applications. Chapter 5 gives many practical examples and applications of care planning using the dental hygiene diagnosis as its guide. Chapter 6 assists the reader in implementing care plans. The final chapter, Evaluation, provides a practical guide and checklist to evaluate care and discusses the issue of quality assurance.

The text is written using many examples and analogies that enable the reader to visualize concepts. At the end of each chapter are exercises that help the reader to self-assess learning. The exercises are designed to build upon each other—as the reader progresses through the book, subsequent chapters contain repeated exercises with additional steps. The answers to the exercises are found in Appendix B.

Appendix A contains four case studies. Each will enable the reader to utilize the skills learned in the text. The cases present assessment information and lead the reader through the process of decision making, formulating the diagnostic statements, selecting dental hygiene interventions, writing expected outcomes of treatment, and care planning. Completion of the case studies will provide the reader with a clear understanding of the dental hygiene process of care.

The authors wish to thank the many colleagues and friends for their help, advice, input, and encouragement, particularly Judith Friedman, RDH, MS, PD, Chair, Department of Dental Hygiene, State University College of Technology at Farmingdale, New York; Margarita Ayala, RDH, MS, Valencia Community College, Florida; and Maureen Lawless-Howes, RDH, MS, Onondaga Community College, New York. We would also like to thank Steve Mruskovic for his help and patience with our diagrams and models and Lois Ulrey at the American Dental Hygienists' Association for her assistance. A special acknowledgment to Joanne Gurenlian for her timely articles and encouragement.

CHAPTER 1

The Dental Hygiene Process of Care

Learning Outcomes

At the completion of the chapter the reader should be able to:

1. List the five phases of the dental hygiene process of care and briefly describe each component
2. List and discuss the six roles and functions of the dental hygienist and their implications to clinical practices as defined by the American Dental Hygienists' Association
3. Describe the three ways the dental hygienist functions within the health care team
4. Briefly describe the benefits of using the dental hygiene process of care for the client, the practitioner, and the profession

INTRODUCTION

Traditionally, many dental hygienists viewed themselves in functional terms, describing their career responsibility in terms of the clinical activities that they performed on a client. When asked what a dental hygienist "does," most hygienists would invariably start with "cleans teeth." The traditional process has been that clients were routinely scheduled for six-month recalls and forty-five-minute appointments. All received approximately the same treatment, and the client expected the practitioner to decide the best course of treatment to keep them in good oral health.

In the late 1960s plaque control programs were developed. This approach to client care revolutionized the practice of dentistry and dental hygiene. The plaque control programs of the 1960s bear little similarity to those of today. Those early programs were highly structured both in timeframe and in the precise education and performance required of the client. The dental professional provided the skill training and education, and the client performed the functions of brushing and flossing. The assessment was based on the client's performance, which required good manipulative skills. What was the norm two or three decades ago is currently considered substandard practice.

Since the inception of the plaque control program, the profession has seen changes that have been evolutionary rather than cataclysmic. However, compared to previous decades, recent technological and pharmacological changes have been rapid and therefore mandate that the profession adapt to changing treatment protocols. Although most of the current treatment modalities are still rooted in plaque control, expanding scientific knowledge of periodontal disease has led to a complex array of diagnostic and treatment options. Our current knowledge of the microflora of the oral cavity has enabled more exact diagnoses. The use of pharmacological interventions has proven to be effective. Technology has created mechanical devices to assist both the client and the practitioner in maintenance, diagnosis, and assessment.

The practice of dental hygiene has moved from an intuitive process that focused mainly on treatment of current conditions to a scientific process that stresses comprehensive assessment to monitor current status and identify potential problem areas. Dental hygiene therapy has progressed to include a complex grouping of assessment indices, treatments, education, and evaluation of therapies.

The current practice of dental hygiene is focused on a conceptual framework of five treatment categories: assessment, dental hygiene diagnosis, planning, implementation, and evaluation, frequently referred to by the acronym *ADPIE*. Earlier models included dental hygiene diagnosis within the assessment phase. However, as dental hygiene care has become more complex and technology has enabled more accurate assessment data, the diagnosis phase has become more essential to good planning. Assessment and planning cannot take place without first defining the direction that the plan will take. Since the five phases are part of an integrated whole and the procedures performed overlap or occur simultaneously, the structure can be termed a *process*. A process is defined as "a series of actions or events; a sequence of operations" (Geddes and Crosset, Ltd., 1990). A series of events can also be *cyclical* (Figure 1.1). Data gathered on a client in the assessment phase is also used in the evaluation phase, which in turn may lead to further assessment, completing and continuing the cycle. The dental hygiene process can also be termed *branching*, with decision-making trees describing alternative treatment and response to therapies (Figure 1.2).

A clinical dental hygienist, practicing in the most up-to-date manner, uses the dental hygiene process to plan treatment tailored to the individual. The complexities of oral health care and the continued changes in technology present challenges to the practitioner. A model that focuses on a process enables the clinician to adjust for changes that occur. Rigid protocols of time and/or treatments are a disservice to the patient and inhibit the practitioner from using knowledge gained in the biomedical and behavioral sciences to determine the course or alternative to treatment. The goal of dental hygiene assessment is to arrive at a reliable and useful judgment based on subjective and objective data. Assessment requires more than learning procedures and techniques. It involves critical thinking and judgment.

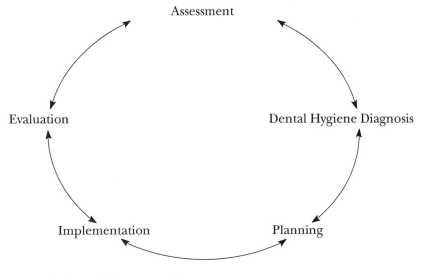

Figure 1.1 *The dental hygiene process cycle*

Societal Influences on Dental Hygiene Practice

Many societal changes have occurred in the past decade that have impacted on the practice of dental hygiene. Clients and their expectations have also changed in the past two decades. Today's health care consumer is more likely to question his or her course of treatment, shop around to find a good match with the health care provider, and expects to participate in treatment decisions. Today's dental client pool consists of more elderly dentate individuals, caries-free children, and culturally diverse patients.

The feminization of the workforce has fostered changes in the family—parents may no longer be solely responsible for their children's daily care. Parents need to ascertain that caregivers are knowledgeable of healthful practices and encourage the adoption of good eating habits and hygiene practices.

Attention to good nutrition is encouraged through recent changes in food labeling and revised daily intake guidelines. Media attention has increased the level of knowledge of healthy food choices. However, busy schedules may force reliance on fast foods or packaged meals that may not meet the standards.

The increased number of individuals utilizing health care insurance may be countered by poor economic conditions and unemployment, which decreases the ability of some to access health care. The recent debates at the national level on health care reform have raised the level of awareness of many health care consumers.

The advent of increased television and print advertising of new over-the-counter oral care products has assisted the profession in making consumers more aware of oral health concerns. However, conflicting claims from manufacturers can lead to misinformation and confusion for the dental professional as well as the consumer. It is the practitioner's responsibility to be cognizant of and knowledgeable about products and be a source of correct and accurate information for the client.

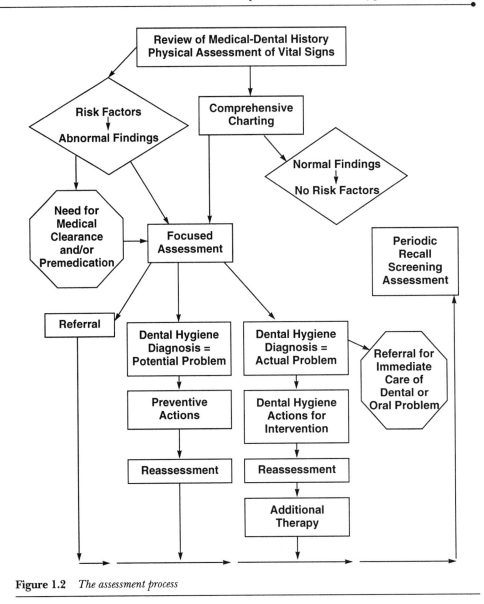

Figure 1.2   *The assessment process*

The practitioner must be aware of the political and/or societal influences on dental practices, at a broad or national level as well as the specific geographic area of one's practice.

Dental Hygiene Practice

Current concepts of dental hygiene practice emphasize the interpersonal, intellectual, and scientific aspects of providing care. The need for a deliberative plan of care, rather than an intuitive or rote performance of activities, is considered the basis of quality care. Comprehensive care, the standard of current practice for today's practicing dental hygienist, requires not only good technical clinical skill, but a myriad of other competencies. The clinician must be skillful in communicating to the client the treatment needs that the assessment data revealed. Knowledge of health education and how to promote behavior change are critical to implementing comprehensive treatment. The clients' medical conditions and use of pharmacological preparations require the hygienist to be aware of their potential impact on dental hygiene care.

In late 1989, the American Dental Hygienists' Association Council on Education recommended that a panel investigate and propose a plan for dental hygiene theory development. The objective was to construct a plan to encourage development of a theoretical framework for dental hygiene practice. The panel agreed that the first step was to define the discipline of dental hygiene, thereby establishing dental hygiene's uniqueness among oral health care professionals. The results of this effort have been approved by the House of Delegates and are included in the 1993 *ADHA Policy Manual* in the section titled Framework for Theory Development.

> The discipline of dental hygiene is the art and science of preventive oral health care including the management of behaviors to prevent oral disease and promote health. Preventive oral health care includes: a) the coordination and delivery of primary preventive oral health educational and clinical services, b) the provision of secondary preventive intervention to prevent further disease and to promote overall health, and c) the facilitation of the client's access to care and implementation of mutually agreed upon oral health care goals. These methods of preventing oral disease and promoting wellness are provided by the dental hygienists in collaboration with the health care team in a variety of settings to all populations—those served, those underserved and those outside the oral health care system. (1993)

Based on the current discipline statement and the current practice of dental hygiene, we can define dental hygiene as an integrated approach recognizing that interaction results from both internal and external forces. Dental hygiene/client interactions are based on *conditions* in which the client enters the dental care system (setting), the *functions* of the dental hygienist in the setting, and the *responsibility* of the dental hygienist in the system. The following model (Figure 1.3) has been developed for the purposes of this book to help define the theory of dental hygiene.

Concepts Defined

Client:	(A) A recipient of dental hygiene care (can refer to individuals or groups); (B) an active participant in dental hygiene process.
Environment:	(A) Economic, psychological, social, and political dimensions affecting optimal health care; (B) clients' and providers' surroundings affecting oral health care.
Health/Oral Health:	The status and oral wellness or illness of the client.

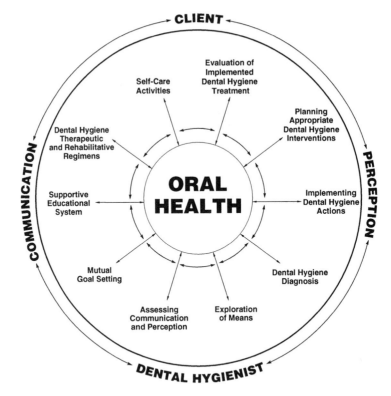

Figure 1.3   *Universal requisites of the dental hygienist—client relationship*

Dental Hygiene Actions: Interventions that a dental hygienist can initiate to promote wellness and to prevent and control oral disease; they involve cognitive, affective, and psychomotor performances.

From this model it can be stated that the dental hygiene process of care is based on a program planning method consisting of assessment, diagnosis, plan development, implementation, and evaluation.

Dental hygiene actions also require skills that incorporate leadership, research, and behavioral principles in the management of the client's health/oral health on the wellness/illness continuum. Dental hygiene actions are implemented in accordance with ethical principles and recognized standards of practice.

DENTAL HYGIENE ROLES AND FUNCTIONS

In 1985, the American Dental Hygienists' Association recognized that the practice of dental hygiene is complex and multifaceted. It was acknowledged that dental hygienists function in many roles: clinician, health educator, researcher, consumer advocate, change agent, and administrator/manager. Each role can be viewed separately, as a researcher working for a company manufacturing dental products or a clinician working in a hospital setting. Alternatively, roles may be viewed as complimentary, performed frequently—even simultaneously—by most practicing hygienists. This book will frequently refer to the dental hygienist as "clinician." It is not our intent to define that role narrowly; rather, it should be understood that the clinician cannot function effectively in one role only. The competent dental hygienist utilizes many abilities and in time skillfully integrates the appropriate knowledge and behaviors required to provide quality dental hygiene care. An example of this is the dental hygienist in a clinical private practice setting, working with each client both as a clinician and an educator. As a change agent, the dental hygienist assists clients in making recommended changes in their behavior and/or assists the practice in making adjustments to treatment protocols. Even in the most limited capacity, the dental hygienist serves as an inventory control manager and a client scheduler, determining the frequency of maintenance visits. The role of researcher may seem remote to many clinicians, but in fact the decisions to implement new treatments, and purchase new products or equipment are usually made after an investigation of alternatives, quality of claims, or personal experience.

Increasing numbers of dental hygienists are conducting applied research in their daily practice with clients by careful objective assessment of treatment protocols. As a consumer advocate, the clinician assures that the client is getting quality products and services for a fair fee by delivering quality care and when recommending dental care products or treatments proven scientifically reliable. This text focuses on the broad definition of clinician—integrating the multiple roles that constitute clinical practice in various settings.

One hallmark of a profession is its ability to assume responsibility for the quality of care that its members provide. In 1985, ADHA published *Standards of Applied Dental Hygiene Practice*. Six standards are listed under the headings of Assessment, Planning, Implementation, and Evaluation. The first two standards define "collection of data, analysis of data," and the "formulation of the dental hygiene diagnosis." The third standard in the planning phase addresses the dental hygiene treatment plan to include "goals and priorities of dental hygiene procedures." Standards 5 and 6 of the implementation phase define the performance of "preventive and therapeutic procedures to prevent or control disease" and "oral health education required to assist the patient in assuming responsibility for their oral health." The final standard refers to evaluation as part of the plan for implementation and as a joint responsibility of the patient and the dental hygienist.

Roles can further be defined as *independent, interdependent,* and *dependent.* Independent functions are those activities that are considered to be within the scope of dental hygiene practice. These actions do not require a direct prescription or order from another professional or authority. It is important to note that each state practice act may limit the performance of some functions, but all recognize the education of the dental hygienist, and by virtue of licensure guarantee a degree of independence of practice even in the supervised setting.

Independent Functions

Independent functions may include, but are not necessarily limited to, the following list. Individuals must be thoroughly familiar with their state practice acts and modify the list as appropriate.

1. Assess the client through comprehensive medical and dental history.

2. Make a physical assessment of vital signs, intra and extra oral evaluation.

3. Complete a comprehensive charting of hard and soft tissues, including plaque; gingival, periodontal, and bleeding indices; caries; restorative charting; descriptions of any oral findings that deviate from the norm; and classification of occlusion.

4. Perform radiographic exposure, processing, mounting, and notation of radiographic findings.

5. Identify those dental hygiene actions that are likely to maintain or restore oral health.

6. Formulate the dental hygiene diagnosis that describes existing or potential oral health problems that the dental hygienist is capable of and licensed to treat.

7. Plan for the dental hygiene treatment of those conditions.

8. Handle case presentation and appointment planning.

9. Implement care designed to motivate and guide, alleviate or eliminate symptoms of disease as required, including all functions legally allowed in the jurisdiction.

10. Educate the client to assume responsibility for his or her oral health.

11. Assist clients to cease using tobacco products.

12. Document and evaluate the client's response to dental hygiene and dental interventions.

13. Refer to other dental or health care team members when indicated.

14. Maintain control of the working environment, including infection control and quality and maintenance of equipment and instruments.

15. Identify and respond to emergency medical situations.

16. Evaluate dental hygiene care products for home and office use.

17. Serve as a resource person for the community on matters pertaining to dental hygiene and prevention of oral disease.

Interdependent Functions

The interdependent functions of the dental hygienist are those carried out in conjunction with other health care team members. The most obvious is the dentist with whom the dental hygienist works. Other dental treatment required by the client must be coordinated and priorities for treatment set with the dental hygiene treatment. In some cases the client will be referred to other dental specialties. At other times the medical history or oral assessment may require collaboration with other health care team members. The dental hygienist is in a unique role as a health professional to observe oral conditions that may be symptomatic of systemic disease. The opportunity to provide oral health education also permits the client to share concerns about a variety of health issues affecting him- or herself or family members. Referrals to other health professionals or agencies can result from those conversations. The dental hygienist who sees his or her scope of practice in the broad sense of a health professional will find many opportunities to help clients avail themselves of other community health resources.

Dependent Functions

Any function legally assigned to the dental hygienist that requires direct supervision, prescription, or dental diagnosis are considered dependent. For example, in New York State the dental hygienist may apply sealants following the dental diagnosis and recommendation. It is a function under direct supervision by New York State legal definition. However, application of fluorides or desensitizing agents that are considered an integral part of the dental hygiene phase of treatment are independent functions.

COMPONENTS OF THE DENTAL HYGIENE PROCESS

The purpose of the dental hygiene process of care is to provide a framework within which the individualized needs of the client can be met. The dental hygiene process is a deliberate, logical, and rational activity performed systematically by the dental hygienist. It is a series of actions that identifies the contributing factors of the current condition. It distinguishes those causative or influencing factors that can be reduced, eliminated, or counteracted by the dental hygienist. The process is designed to provide dental hygiene therapy that will maintain or restore the client's optimal oral health.

Throughout the process the practitioner makes use of a comprehensive knowledge base to assess the client's health status, make judgments and diagnoses, plan and implement care, and evaluate the progress and results of these interventions.

The five interacting components introduced previously are outlined below with various steps. These will be elaborated on further in this section.

1. **Assessment**
   a. data collection
   b. documentation (charting)
2. **Dental Hygiene Diagnosis**
   a. analysis/synthesis of data
   b. diagnostic statements
3. **Planning**
   a. priorities
   b. goals and objectives
   c. change strategies
   d. dental hygiene treatment plan
4. **Implementation**
5. **Evaluation**

Assessment

Assessment is the first phase of the dental hygiene process. It is a continuous process that collects both objective and subjective data needed to provide care. The data should be comprehensive and multifocal, representing a variety of sources. Activities are based on gathering information regarding the client's present state of health for the purpose of identifying the client's needs, problems, concerns, and/or human responses. Data are collected in a systematic fashion, utilizing the health/dental history, intra and extra oral examination, restorative chart, gingival assessment, periodontal evaluation, oral health indices, laboratory results, and other sources. It is a dynamic process with changes occurring as more data are collected and the client's condition alters.

Subjective data is obtained by observation and interaction with the client. The collection of such data requires well developed interpersonal skills on the part of the practitioner. These data can be obtained from the client, family, or caretakers. It consists of the client's signs and symptoms, feelings, perception of health care, value of oral health, and the perceived management of those concerns.

Objective data is measurable and includes physical and oral assessment. It requires the practitioner to have good technical skills and consistency in the language of descriptive statements used from client to client. Results of laboratory tests, records, observations of other health team members all form a part of the objective database. Since data collection is an ongoing process, an appropriate method of documentation must be devised.

Dental Hygiene Diagnosis

This phase critically analyzes and interprets the data collected during the assessment phase, thereby identifying the client's needs. Many diagnostic models have been identified and used in the health professions. Medicine and dentistry focus on the diagnosis and treatment of disease; nursing focuses on the health functioning of the individual and describes the actual or potential health problems that nurses are able and licensed to treat (Hickey, 1990). Accepted nursing diagnoses do not permit identification of a disease such as diabetes, but identify the potential problems that the client may encounter related to the symptoms of the disease, such as "potential for impaired wound healing." The dental hygiene diagnosis as presented in this text and by other authors is patterned on the diagnostic models found in other health professions.

Gurenlian (1990) describes the process of dental hygiene diagnostic decision making as involving six steps:

1. Initial review
2. Hypothesis formulation
3. Inquiry strategy
4. Problem synthesis
5. Diagnostic decision making
6. Learning from the process

The initial review gives a broad picture of the client and clues to the hypothesis formulation, which identifies the possible labels that might be applied to the client's health problems. Inquiry strategy helps to focus or test the original hypothesis. Questioning, lab tests, and radiographs are examples of assessment procedures that would assist the clinician in formulating the hypothesis. Problem synthesis summarizes the facts and eliminates the useless or extraneous information. The fifth step is formulating the diagnostic statement, and finally learning from the process takes place over time by reviewing the elements.

Dental hygienists by virtue of their education have learned that diseases have certain defining characteristics. To avoid the use of all reference to disease entities, as the nursing model of diagnosis does, would be extremely limiting to the formulation of the dental hygiene diagnosis. As an example, during the hypothesis formulation stage, the clinician would review the conditions or diseases that the assessment data identified as possibilities. A client has multiple painful ulcers. The hygienist may consider herpes, recurrent aphthous ulcers, or contact stomatitis as possible causes. The hygienist would then consider what further information needs to be gathered before focusing on the specific cause of the client's problem. Once the problem is identified, the hygienist decides its likely cause. Following the diagnostic stage, the clinician would then start to plan for care that will ameliorate the present condition or avoid future attacks.

Another model recently introduced to dental hygiene is the human needs conceptual model, by Darby and Walsh, which is based on the nursing model that evaluates client function. Because historically dental hygienists have focused on client behaviors as they relate to oral disease rather than on oral disease itself, they selected the human needs theory and applied that to the four paradigm concepts of client, environment, health/oral health, and dental hygiene actions. This topic is covered in more detail in Chapter 4.

The dental hygiene diagnostic model proposed in this text is also based on the nursing model, but does not impose the restriction of avoiding disease terminology. For instance, the nursing model would strictly prohibit the use of such terms as "gingivitis" or "periodontitis type II." The authors believe that eliminating all disease terminology would be too limiting to be beneficial to the client. The limitation espoused in this text is to those conditions that are treatable by the dental hygienist. Dental caries, for instance, would be a dental diagnosis since its treatment would require restorations. Potential for decalcification in the future, however, would fall within the dental hygienist's scope of practice, since the behaviors that led to the current problem could be altered through education, behavior change strategies, and preventive therapies.

Diagnosis is a two-step process—analysis/synthesis of data and the development of diagnostic statements. *Data analysis and synthesis* identifies conditions, problems, and concerns and compares them to standards of care and known successful interventions. The association of the problems, etiology, current signs and symptoms, the client's behavioral patterns and oral health concerns all form the basis of the dental hygiene diagnosis.

The second step is the *development of diagnostic statements*. The diagnosis must be client-centered, specific, and accurate. It should be a clear, concise statement describing the existing condition and possible etiology. The dental hygiene diagnostic statement must reflect only those oral health concerns that can be treated by the dental hygienist. It provides the basis on which the dental hygiene treatment plan is designed, implemented, and evaluated. The dental hygiene diagnosis differs from the dental diagnosis, since a dental diagnosis refers to the identification of a disease process or entity and the dental hygiene diagnosis identifies the client's actual or potential response to the disease process. The dental hygiene diagnosis identifies those aspects of the client's care for which the hygienist would be responsible. It may be obvious that a client's maxillary full denture needs relining or reconstruction. The dental hygiene diagnosis would focus on educating the client to recognize the need and benefit, whereas the dental diagnosis would address the relining or reconstruction. Should the client accede to the need, the hygienist may be called upon to take impressions for study models. This interdependent function would then become part of the subsequent care plan.

Planning

The planning phase develops strategies to meet the unique needs of the client as identified in the dental hygiene diagnosis. The planning phase consists of several steps:

1. Establishing priorities for the identified needs
2. Setting outcomes with the client to meet the established needs
3. Developing dental hygiene care plans that will lead to the achievement of the proposed outcomes

The conditions diagnosed must be put in priority order and the goals, objectives, and strategies must be mutually agreed upon by the client and the dental hygienist. Care plan goals are expected client outcomes that are stated in broad terms. Several objectives may be written to achieve each goal. They should include measurable criteria that enable assessment of the steps to be taken to achieve the goal. Objectives should reflect a realistic resolution of the diagnosis and be written within the client's capabilities and limitations. The choice of a strategy to achieve the desired outcome is integral to the formulation of the goals. The strategy chosen is based upon the anticipated effectiveness in achieving the desired outcome, the benefits and risks to the client and the available resources, including time, equipment, finances, facilities, and family support systems.

The dental hygiene treatment plan is written in terms of the client and practitioner's behaviors for each objective and the time period in which they will be accomplished. The treatment plan should be stated in concise terms so that it is easily understandable and with an appropriate sequence of treatments that progress in an orderly, beneficial manner.

Implementation

This phase consists of the implementation of the dental hygiene interventions necessary to achieve the outcomes defined in the planning stage. The activities to be performed by the client and practitioner or others identified in the treatment plan are conducted in this phase. Interdisciplinary coordination of treatment therapies (oral and systemic) must be considered to provide optimal care. In addition, all treatment must be properly documented and evaluated.

Evaluation

Evaluation is an ongoing process. While implementing the treatment plan, valuative judgments must be made that describe the client's responses—both physical and behavioral—to each phase of the dental hygiene treatment. This formative evaluation provides continual data that may be used to change or modify the treatment plan. Evaluation must compare the client's current status with the baseline data and progress, or lack thereof, towards the stated goals.

IMPLICATIONS OF THE DENTAL HYGIENE PROCESS

The terms "quality care" and "current concepts" of dental hygiene are frequently used. Their meanings, however, can be interpreted in different ways and may vary for different geographic areas and change over a period of time. Lee and Jones (1933) defined good health care as "practiced and taught by the recognized leaders of the profession at a given period of time . . . ". They further propose eight "articles of faith":

Good health care

1. is limited to the practice of rational medicine based on the health sciences.
2. emphasizes prevention.
3. requires intelligent cooperation between the lay public and the practitioners of scientific medicine.
4. treats the individual as a whole.
5. maintains a close and continuing personal relation between provider and patient.
6. is coordinated with social welfare work.
7. coordinates all types of health services.
8. implies application of all necessary services of modern, scientific medicine to the needs of the people.

What is interesting about the previous work is that is was published in 1933. The dental hygiene process fulfills all of the articles. It is the essence of quality care. The process serves as a model and is therefore in itself timeless. New techniques, procedures, and instrumentation or equipment are inserted into the process as additions or replacements.

Implications for the Client

The use of a systematic method of providing dental hygiene therapy improves the quality of care. The dental hygiene process provides a model for a carefully engineered and monitored plan. It provides the client with three fundamental components:

Information. Assessment of the individual reveals objective and subjective data of the current or potential condition. It provides the client with factual information. It permits a comparison to previous visits and forms the database for further evaluation.

Alternatives. Collaboration of client and practitioner allows a sharing of views, opinions, and/or attitudes of the alternative diagnosis and treatment options. Consideration is given to the client's capacity for change and ability to accept financial and time management responsibilities.

Preferences. Preferences for treatment must be negotiated between the client and practitioner. The practitioner must explicitly represent the outcome of treatment, acknowledging the value the client has placed on the outcome. Since the client may have little experience in the decision-making process, the practitioner should guide, but not determine, the final decision.

Inherent in the process is the opportunity for the client to participate in all phases of treatment. As assessment takes place, the client is made aware of the conditions that are present and the actual or potential problems that those conditions may yield. The care plan should be seen as a negotiated contract between two individuals with each agreeing to perform certain tasks to a greater or lesser degree than the other. The client is also a partner in the evaluation of the outcome, both of the part that they assumed and that which the clinician provided.

Informed consent, which enables the client to be part of treatment decisions, is an integral part of practice. It is the legal reason for presenting a care plan to the client. The client's condition must be described accurately in terms that are understandable. The client needs to have time to question and confirm his or her understanding. The likely outcome of treatment must be described, as well as any risks or negative side effects. The client should be informed of any alternative treatments or the likely outcome of refusing treatment. Estimates of cost and time should be addressed. Accurate and detailed documentation of client care activities and interactions are required for legal purposes and to ensure the continuity of care.

Implications for the Practitioner

The dental hygiene process of providing client care increases career satisfaction and encourages professional growth. Miller (1991), in a study of dental hygienists' leaving the profession, cited "lack of decision-making opportunities and to a lesser degree, lack of opportunities for collaboration with employers," as important reasons. Each client is seen as an individual requiring innovation and creativity in solving problems and planning for care. The rewards resulting from this approach affect the clinician as well as the client. Meaningful dental hygienist/client relationships develop with increased success and fewer failures and frustration. The application of the process encourages the development of skills in interpersonal relationships as well as technical and clinical expertise.

Implications for the Profession

The dilemma of defining the scope of practice is not unique to dental hygiene. Nurses, physical therapists, and dieticians are some who have struggled to define their roles and professions. The complexity of health care and the integration of treatment makes clearly defined duties assigned to one profession and denied to another a task that would ultimately result in fragmentation of treatment and disservice to clients.

It is important to recognize the body of knowledge of each profession. In an educated and technological society, consumers are not content to have untrained people provide them with medical or dental treatment. Professions such as dental hygiene focus on one segment of the total oral health care picture. A general dentist is educated in all segments of oral health care to some degree. That practitioner may extract teeth, construct prosthetic appliances, and perform root canal therapy in daily practice. However, that same practitioner probably refers clients to the oral surgeon, prosthodontist, and endodontist for those cases deemed complicated or beyond the scope of that individual's practice. That same dentist may employ a dental hygienist because he or she recognizes that the dental hygienist has the skill, knowledge, and ability to perform nonsurgical periodontal therapy and periodontal maintenance therapy for the clients of that practice, and has the scope of practice to provide all aspects of dental hygiene care. The profession of dentistry and dental hygiene, as well as the legal jurisdiction of that locale, has further assured both the employer and the consumer of the services that the individual has the education, knowledge, and skill to perform. It becomes incumbent upon that dental hygienist to assess each client carefully and decide when a case is beyond the scope of dental hygiene treatment and needs to be referred either to the dentist within that general practice or to the periodontal specialist, either of whom may provide more complicated surgical procedures.

The issue of scope of practice is both a professional issue and a personal one. The profession through practice acts, accreditation, and state and national board examinations has defined a body of knowledge and allowable functions for the profession of dental hygiene. Through personal study, experience, and continuing education, the individual defines his or her own scope of practice. Those limits may revolve around a central core or to the limits that are professionally and legally permitted. Two hygienists working in the same dental practice may view their scope of practice differently because of their experience, education, or personality. These perceptions need to be discussed and negotiated so the clients of the practice receive equitable treatment and each clinician has the opportunity to practice to the limits of his or her ability.

Summary

The dental hygiene process of care is a model for providing systematic, individualized, quality dental hygiene care. The process is composed of five components: assessment, diagnosis, planning, implementation, and evaluation, each dependent and interdependent on the other. Mastery of this process will enable the dental hygienist to focus on decision making and evaluate treatment based on client need. It will also provide a mechanism to help define our professional role and scope of practice.

REFERENCES

American Dental Hygienists' Association. (1985). *Standards of applied dental hygiene practice.* Chicago: Author.

American Dental Hygienists' Association. (1993). *Policy manual framework for theory development.* Chicago: Author.

Geddes and Crosset, Ltd. (1990). *Webster's new dictionary and thesaurus, concise edition.* New Lanark, Scotland: Author.

Gurenlian, J.R. (1990). Diagnostic Decision Making. In I.R. Woodall (Ed.), *Comprehensive dental hygiene care* (pp. 361–370). St. Louis, MO: Mosby.

Hickey, P.W. (1990). *Nursing process handbook.* St. Louis, MO: Mosby.

Lee, R.J., & Jones, L.W. (1933). *The fundamentals of good medical care.* Chicago: University of Chicago Press.

Miller, D. (1991). An investigation into attrition of dental hygienists from the work force. *Journal of Dental Hygiene, 65,* 25–31.

Exercise 1.1　Roles of the Dental Hygienist

Either by yourself or with a small group, describe the various activities or procedures that a dental hygienist might perform in the six roles for the following practice settings. It is possible that not all the roles for each practice setting will be filled.

	Private Dental Practice	Nursing Home Clinic	Dental Product Sales Representative	Research Consultant
Clinician				
Health Educator				
Researcher				
Consumer Advocate				
Change Agent[1]				
Administrator/ Manager				

1 Change agent is generally meant as one who works within the system to change policies, procedures, or legislation.

Exercise 1.2　Changing Times

Investigate the following topics, using a textbook with multiple editions or journal articles. Determine what, if any, changes have occurred over the last decade or two. Use the most current edition available or one from the 1990s, then compare to one from the 1980s, 1970s, or 1960s.

1. Sterilization/infection control
2. Sealants
3. Polishing tooth surfaces
4. Plaque microbiology
5. Irrigation
6. Fluoride application

Some questions to help focus your comparisons:

a. What major differences did you note?

b. How did the information change?

c. Were there any changes in protocols or techniques?

d. What similarities were there?

e. What are the implications of this comparison?

Exercise 1.3   Functioning as Part of the Team

Using the following list, identify those functions that are Independent (I), Interdependent (IT), and Dependent (D). Use your own State Practice Act as a guide.

_____ 1. Exposure of radiographs

_____ 2. Nutritional counseling

_____ 3. Providing patient information on a smoking cessation program in the community

_____ 4. Taking blood pressure

_____ 5. Using a periodontal index

_____ 6. Sealant application

_____ 7. Classroom presentation during Dental Health Month

_____ 8. Medical history indicating hip prosthesis

_____ 9. Prescription of prophylactic antibiotic

_____ 10. Referral of patient to periodontist

_____ 11. Use of phase contrast microscope

_____ 12. Coordination of patient's dental hygiene therapy with the prosthodontist

_____ 13. Establishing the protocol for the sterilization of dental hygiene instruments

Exercise 1.4   Knowledge Test of Process

Match the phase of the dental hygiene process in Column I with the description in Column II.

Column I	***Column II***

_____ 1. Assessment

    A. Data analysis and identification of client's actual or potential health problem

_____ 2. Dental Hygiene Diagnosis

    B. Examination of the client to determine if the desired outcomes have been achieved

_____ 3. Planning

    C. Collection of subjective and objective data

_____ 4. Implementation

    D. Development of desired outcomes and determination of strategies to achieve them

_____ 5. Evaluation

    E. Coordination of dental and dental hygiene therapies

CHAPTER 2

Assessment

Learning Outcomes

At the completion of the chapter the reader should be able to:

1. Identify the two components of a comprehensive dental hygiene assessment
2. Differentiate between subjective and objective data
3. Explain the importance of each data collection category in the assessment phase
4. Recognize the importance of the client interview to validate assessment findings
5. Compare and contrast data collected during the initial client appointment with data collected at future appointments

INTRODUCTION

The assessment phase of the dental hygiene process of care can be defined as an organized, systematic process of collecting data from a variety of sources to evaluate the health status of a client. It provides a foundation that promotes the delivery of quality *individualized* care. Accurate, complete assessment is necessary for the identification of dental hygiene diagnoses, development of treatment plans, implementation of interventions, and evaluation of outcomes.

The initial assessment enables the dental hygienist to accumulate comprehensive baseline data (see Table 2.1) about the client's overall health as well as his or her oral health conditions. Baseline data collection begins as soon as the client enters the health care setting and continues throughout the first appointment. This initial appointment usually requires a minimum of one to one and one-half hours to collect data accurately and assess the client's condition systematically.

Table 2.1 • **BASELINE DATA COLLECTED DURING THE ASSESSMENT PHASE**

SUBJECTIVE DATA	General Information
	Personal Profile
	Dental History
	Medical History
OBJECTIVE DATA	Extra Oral Examination
	Intra Oral Examination
	Dental Examination
	Periodontal Examination
	Oral Hygiene Evaluation
	Radiographic Examination
	Laboratory Tests
	Clinical Photography

Subsequent assessments validate the existence of previously identified conditions and documents the client's progress towards the established goals. Since assessment is a continuous process, subsequent data enables the dental hygienist to identify additional problems that may have developed as a result of the disease process or noncompliance. Subsequent assessment is accomplished by comparing current information (data) to previously acquired baseline data.

PREPROCESS

Prior to the implementation of the dental hygiene process of care, the dental hygienist must acquire a scientific knowledge base and a variety of interpersonal and technical skills. These fundamental principles are usually sequenced so that by the time a dental hygiene student is in his or her second clinical semester they can easily be applied to the process of care.

Knowledge

The process of assessment requires more than learning procedures and techniques. It involves critical thinking and judgment. Therefore, the dental hygienist must possess an extensive body of knowledge from a variety of disciplines, including both physical and behavioral sciences. The dental hygienist is expected to master basic concepts of anatomy, physiology, pharmacology, chemistry, microbiology, psychology, and sociology. The components of this scientific base allow the dental hygienist to make initial assessments of the client's state of health. Such a body of knowledge also forms the basis for recognition of change during subsequent assessments.

The dental hygienist's knowledge base must also include the fundamentals of problem solving, analysis, and decision making. The dental hygienist must be able to analyze assessment data, recognize significant relationships among data, develop valid conclusions, and subsequently make sound dental hygiene judgments that contribute to the client's progress.

Skills

A variety of skills are necessary for the dental hygienist to complete an effective assessment. These skills are related to the knowledge base and may be both interpersonal and technical in nature.

Interpersonal skills are important during all phases of the dental hygiene process but are particularly critical to a successful assessment, which requires extensive communication and interaction with the client. How an individual interacts with others using communication to promote effective relationships is the definition of interpersonal skill. The model for effective interpersonal communication is:

$$\text{Message Formed} \longrightarrow \text{Message Sent} \longrightarrow \text{Message Received}$$

This basic model is, however, far from simple. Just as it is the basis for understanding, it can also be the basis for misunderstanding.

The clinician's use of language, nonverbal behavior, and listening skills are an important part of effective communication. The ability to assess the client's knowledge and behavior without portraying him or her as deficient or inadequate is a skill to be cultivated. There are numerous texts addressing the topics of communication and interpersonal skills for the health professional that should be consulted for a more thorough review of the topics. However, since the ability to transmit accurate and timely information, identify needs, and influence behavior change is the basis for successful treatment outcomes, a brief discussion of communication skills follows.

Most client visits begin with a medical history. This may be a brief review or a lengthy interview depending upon the protocols. In either case, the questioning begins soon after the initial pleasantries and introductions are accomplished.

Each of us has gone through the experience of having to describe experiences, justify actions, or recall details of past activities. For some, the recollection will be easy and pleasant, for others it will cause anxiety or produce anger. The fact gathering should be accomplished with open-ended questions that seek information without judgment. The manner in which an interview is conducted sets the tone for the relationship. If the client feels he or she is undergoing an interrogation rather than an interview, his or her attitude will be negative. A skillful interviewer gets impressions and feelings of events, rather than just the facts.

An interview involves complex communication and requires the dental hygienist to process the information received, not merely record an answer. The function of the interview is to collect information that will ultimately be used in the decision-making process. It includes the medical-dental history, as well as the current preventive health behavior of the client, and his or her attitudes and values toward health. The dental hygiene diagnosis and treatment plan are based on assessing and interpreting human responses in attitudes as well as the objective data recorded from various charting and indices. Enelow and Swisher (1979) identify three general characteristics of the successful interview.

1. The interviewer's behavior should encourage communication. The interview should start with open-ended, nonjudgmental questions. "Tell me about your

usual home care routine" or "How have you been getting along since your last visit?" invite open, honest responses. More specific questions can then follow to clarify answers. Give the client time to answer without feeling pressured or embarrassed by the interview.

2. The interviewer should give attention to the client's non-verbal behavior as well as his or her story. What the client doesn't say may be as important as what is said. The SIT principle is proposed by Chamber and Abrams (1986) to help read nonverbal communication.

    a. Place the gesture, expression, or voice characteristic in the total **S**ituation.

    b. **I**nterpret its meaning tentatively, as in a hypothesis.

    c. **T**est to verify that your interpretation is meaningful.

As an example, one widely held notion is that a crossed-arm pose means the individual is "closed" or defensive. Asking the client "How do you feel?" or "Are you comfortable?" may elicit responses that assure you the client is merely assuming a comfortable position.

3. The interviewer should move through a cycle of information seeking that begins with low use of authority and proceeds to progressively greater authority.

The open-ended, nonjudgmental questions should begin the interview, since they elicit information without threat. In the dental office this is critical. Many clients are fearful or apprehensive about treatment. Others come in feeling guilty about their own poor preventive behavior. "What brought you here today?" establishes a chief complaint without talking about "What's wrong with you?" If the client won't share information, or the verbal information is not congruent with the nonverbal behavior or the clinical signs and symptoms, then the practitioner must point this out by drawing the person's attention to the observed signs and symptoms or behavior in a reasonable, non-argumentative manner. Asking direct questions for specific details may be necessary.

The interview also gives the practitioner the opportunity to establish rapport and begin to gain insight into the client's attitude, values, and preventive health behaviors. The client should be seated upright and placed at eye level during the interview. Once the hygienist picks up an instrument and the client's mouth is opened, the client may feel powerless to communicate. Having established a concerned, empathetic, and nonjudgmental attitude during the initial portion of the assessment interview will enhance the hygienist's opportunity to comment upon conditions that are present as the oral assessment continues. Nonverbal behavior of both hygienist and client become very important at this point. The practitioner must project professional expertise and acceptance of the current conditions.

Technical skills associated with the assessment phase involve specific techniques and procedures that allow the dental hygienist to collect data. Some are associated with the use of equipment, such as stethoscopes, sphygmomanometers, explorers, and periodontal probes, while other technical skills involve performance procedures, such as palpation of lymph nodes and oral tissues, or tactile sensitivity for the detection of calculus deposits and tooth irregularities. Both types of technical skills are required for an accurate, complete assessment.

COMPONENTS OF THE ASSESSMENT PHASE

Assessment consists of two basic components: *comprehensive data collection* and *documentation*. Data collection is comprised of the medical/oral history and a complete clinical examination, including data from radiographs, diagnostic tests, and photographs. All data collected must be documented in the client's chart for easy access during analysis and interpretation. Although there are no short cuts to obtaining an accurate assessment, the amount and complexity of information collected is dependent on the client's condition. It is obvious that modifications to data collection are in order when dealing with children, fully edentulous clients, or others with special situations, problems, or difficulties. Therefore, for the purposes of this book, we will be concentrating on the characteristics of a typical adult dental client.

The completion of an accurate assessment requires an organized, systematic approach to ensure that all pertinent information is collected and recorded. Table 2.2 identifies a suggested step-by-step guide to the assessment phase. A systematic approach toward data collection will minimize errors and increase confidence. As previously mentioned, it takes time to be precise. The time spent should be viewed as an investment. The benefits reaped will be counted in increased compliance and patient satisfaction.

Table 2.2 • **ASSESSMENT GUIDE**

STEP 1:	Collect subjective information
	—General information
	—Personal profile data
	—Medical/dental history
STEP 2:	Identify any potential or actual finding that would stop the assessment process
STEP 3:	Obtain client consent
STEP 4:	Collect objective information
	—Extra oral exam
	—Intra oral exam
	—Dental exam
	—Periodontal exam
	—Oral hygiene evaluation
	—Radiographic survey
	—Laboratory tests
	—Photographs
STEP 5:	Analyze findings
STEP 6:	Interpret findings
STEP 7:	Continue with ongoing or follow-up assessments

DATA COLLECTION

Types of Data

Data collected by the dental hygienist during the assessment phase includes subjective data, objective data, historical data, and current data. A combination of all four types is the basis for an accurate and complete assessment.

Subjective data might be described as the individual's opinion of a situation rather than substantiated fact. This information is determined by interaction and communication with the client. Subjective data are frequently obtained during personal profile, medical/dental history, and chief complaint. This type of data includes the client's perceptions, feelings, and ideas about his or her personal health status. For example, if a client states "I have pain on the left side whenever I have something cold to drink," or "My gums bleed," they are giving subjective data.

Additional types of subjective data may be supplied by sources other than the client such as family, caretakers, and other members of the health care team. Knowledge of the community or geographic area may also contribute to the database. Availability of public health care programs and the level of fluoridation in the community are some examples. This is the assessment phase and the more information collected, the easier it is for the dental hygienist to make a diagnosis and plan for treatment.

In contrast, *objective data* is data that can be externally measured or evaluated. Examples of objective data in dental hygiene are found in the clinical examination and include the components of vital signs, extra oral exam, intra oral exam, restorative charting, periodontal evaluation, oral hygiene evaluation, radiographs, and laboratory tests. Objective data can be easily measured numerically or descriptively and compared when necessary. Comparisons of objective data form the basis for determining the client's progress. Measurements collected at the initial visit are identified as baseline data and are usually used to make comparisons with measurements following treatment.

Research directs the degree of importance of specific types of objective data in dental hygiene and other health care professions. For example, the nonspecific plaque hypothesis (Theilade, 1986) stated that there is a direct relationship between the amount of plaque present and the degree of gingival or periodontal disease. Based on this finding the dental plaque index became a valuable tool in assessing the client's disease status and home care practices. However, as research progressed and the specific plaque hypothesis was postulated (Slots, 1986), the objective data emphasis shifted from plaque accumulation to the identification of plaque microorganisms for assessing disease status. Industry recognized the need to identify the types of microorganisms and pathogen tests became available. This example demonstrates how technological advances change the practice of dental hygiene.

Objective data encompasses a large portion of client assessment and many dental corporations have developed specialized equipment to facilitate its collection. The automated periodontal probe is considered a fairly new piece of equipment that is gaining considerable attention. The Interprobe™ (Bausch and Lomb Oral Health Care Division, Tucker, GA) and the Florida probe™ (Florida Probe Corp., Gainesville, FL) are two automated probing systems on the market. These systems assist in the measurement of pocket probing depth, loss of attachment, and gingival recession with the help of a computer. The clinician still needs the skill of tactile sensitivity to place the probe properly; however, the system measures the identified structure and records the data in a computer base that generates a hard copy for the client's chart.

Another consideration when describing data is the element of time. In this context, data may be classified as historical or current (Bellack and Bamford, 1984). *Historical data* involves information about events that have occurred prior to the present, such as tooth extraction, root canal therapy, and periodontal surgery. In contrast, *current data* refers to events that are occurring in the present, such as elevated blood pressure, tooth sensitivity, and gingival bleeding. Historical and current data assist in establishing timeframes for events and substantiate the occurrence of findings.

A combination of subjective, objective, historical, and current data may be used to verify problems, identify discrepancies, and validate progress. Frequently the different types of data collected support each other, as in the case of the client who has pain when drinking something cold. The client's subjective statement "It feels like a cavity when I drink something cold" was supported by the dental hygienist's objective finding of a broken tooth. Exercise 2.1 at the end of this chapter is designed to assist you in recognizing the different types of data collected during the assessment phase.

Data Collection Categories

The following discussion will be limited to what is considered the minimum standard of practice for what information should be included in a typical adult client assessment. There are numerous dental hygiene textbooks available designed to give specific information on each of the following topics. The reader is strongly encouraged to consult these texts for a more thorough understanding.

GENERAL INFORMATION

General information is collected for client identification as well as insight into the client's state of health. It includes client's full name, address, home and business phone numbers, occupation, age, sex, race, marital status, party to contact in case of an emergency, third party payment (insurance company), and the name and phone number of the client's physician. All of this general information is usually provided by the client on a form that is filled out upon arrival and updated as necessary.

PERSONAL PROFILE

The client's personal profile is obtained via subjective evaluation and is collected to gain valuable information regarding the client's individual characteristics. Some areas to explore include the following:

1. Attitude—How does the client respond to the dental setting? Is the client apprehensive, hostile, and noncommunicative or is he or she relaxed, friendly, and responsive?

2. Value of treatment—Does the client desire preventive therapy to avoid emergency situations?

3. Family history—Is there a family history of periodontitis? caries? oral cancer? genetic oral diseases?

4. Socioeconomic status—What is the client's lifestyle? Sometimes this finding will direct treatment options.

5. Dental beliefs—Does the client have any dental beliefs that are considered myths, such as you lose a tooth every time you have a baby?

DENTAL HISTORY

The dental history includes such information as the chief complaint, present illness, past dental problems or treatment, oral habits, and dietary profile. This information is also collected subjectively via a written form and an interview with the client. The information obtained as part of the dental history will influence the approach towards future treatment.

Chief Complaint.   The chief complaint is a simple statement identifying why the client is seeking treatment. Although this may seem easy, for many clients it is difficult to verbalize problems. As a dental hygienist it is important not to supply the answers for the client. The best way to help a client express his or her concerns is to listen and respond reflectively. In other words, restate the client's concerns without changing the interpretation. For example, the client states "I'm worried sick about the pain I am experiencing. I hope I'm not going to lose any teeth." The appropriate reflective response should be "It's frightening when you don't know what's causing the pain. You tend to suspect the worst" (Ingersol, 1982). Reflective responding is a communicative technique used to comfort the client and clarify subjective information.

Present Dental Illness.   The present dental illness is the history of the chief complaint. It includes, in chronological order, the events from onset to the present. During this portion of the data collection phase the dental hygienist can probe the client to gain more specific information concerning his or her condition. The focus of the probing questions might be the nature and type of pain or sensitivity. Sometimes clients are not aware of a present dental illness; in this case, the focus of questioning would be to verify health.

Past Dental and Dental Hygiene History.   This category includes information concerning past dental problems as well as past dental treatment. Identification of the client's dental care history should be obtained to provide insight into the client's dental care values.

Some questions to consider are:

1. Tell me about the reason for your last dental/dental hygiene visit (Was it for routine dental treatment, prophylaxis and examination, or emergency treatment?).

2. How long has it been since you had preventive therapy? How do you feel about that length of time?

3. Do you follow a routine periodontal maintenance program?

4. When was the last time you had radiographs taken? Was it a full mouth series?

5. What type of home care procedures do you perform? Do you use any type of mouth rinse? What kind of toothpaste do you use?

In addition, questions should be asked to determine how the client feels (subjectively) about the past dental problems and/or treatment encountered. Statements related to previous extractions, periodontal treatment, orthodontic treatment, and endodontic treatment are also important. Past dental/dental hygiene experiences can provide the dental hygienist with clues to form the foundation for successful treatment outcomes.

Oral Habits.   Questions relating to the client's oral habits may provide information to substantiate the present dental illness. For example, the client states, "My mouth aches when I wake up in the morning." Upon questioning the client about his oral habits, he states that he used to wear a mouth guard at night because he would grind his teeth when he slept. Nocturnal bruxism is an oral habit that can cause the muscles of mastication to work overtime. The overworking of these muscles produce a tired, aching feeling in the jaws. Follow-up questions about why the mouth guard isn't currently being used should then be asked.

Dietary Profile.   As dental hygienists, we have been educated regarding nutritional health; however, we may not have sufficient knowledge to intervene when complex nutritional deficits exist. Therefore, the focus of a client's dietary profile is primarily to gather information and direct obvious problems beyond the scope of the dental hygienist's expertise to the appropriate medical professional. If the client has an excessive amount of sucrose (refined carbohydrates) in his or her diet, and the frequency of consumption is high, then a potential caries problem may exist. Since this is directly related to our scope of practice, we can intervene by suggesting ways to alter the client's dietary habits to maintain good dental health. In addition, dietary deficiencies and disorders, such as bulimia and anorexia, might be recognized. In this type of situation, medical assistance should be offered to the client by directing him or her to the appropriate medical resource.

MEDICAL HISTORY

The medical history is one of the most important parts of the assessment phase. An accurate medical history will decrease the potential of a medical/dental office emergency and will provide the dental hygienist with pertinent information to guide treatment options with the client's best interests in mind. The medical history must be obtained at the client's first appointment and updated periodically. The following information should be included in the history:

1. Client's general health. When was the client's last physical examination? Is the client presently under the care of a physician? If so, for what condition? What medications (prescription or nonprescription) is the client presently taking?

2. Allergies and sensitivity. Has the client ever had an adverse reaction to medication, food, pollen, or anything else? If so, what type of reaction occurred?

3. Review of the systems. A thorough review of each body system is an attempt to uncover undiagnosed diseases and to be sure all relevant information is collected. The following list of body systems should be reviewed.

> Head, ears, eyes, nose, and throat
>
> Respiratory
>
> Cardiovascular
>
> Gastrointestinal
>
> Genitourinary
>
> Muscles, bones, and joints
>
> Central nervous system
>
> Endocrine
>
> Hematologic

Table 2.3 contains some common medical problems that interfere with or contraindicate dental/dental hygiene treatment.

In many busy dental offices it is common practice to have the client fill out the medical/dental history in the reception room, independently, at the start of the appointment. A number of studies have identified that the self-report health history questionnaire is not reliable. Brady and Martinoff (1980) indicated that 30 percent of the more than 2,000 clients they screened reported they were in good health, when in fact their health was not good, using accepted norms in the Patient Classification System by the American Academy of Anesthesiology. Another study (Fenlon and McCartlan, 1992) reported many dental clients did not think their past medical history had anything to do with dental treatment, including reporting cardiovascular disease, adverse drug reactions, and relevant drug therapies.

Since the dental hygienist is frequently the first professional in the office the client sees, either as a new client or for maintenance visits, the dental hygienist must accept the responsibility of validating the health history. If the system used is self-report, then additional questioning of the client is required to verify the information, starting first with open-ended and continuing with more probing questions. A study of over 4500 dental hygienists nationwide indicated that 66 percent of the dental hygienists surveyed were solely responsible for updating the medical history for recall clients and 15 percent for new clients. Only 6 percent reported that the dentist took sole responsibility for the medical history with new clients and a very low 0.6 percent with recall clients (Benicewicz & Metzger, 1989). Therefore, it is imperative that the dental hygienist thoroughly review the client's medical history and identify conditions that may interfere with or contraindicate treatment. Additionally, research demonstrates that the dentist's involvement almost always occurs after dental hygiene services are completed (Boyer and Gupta, 1990).

The following section of data collection refers to the clinical examination, which includes such examinations as the extra oral exam, the intra oral exam, the

Table 2.3 • COMMON MEDICAL CONDITIONS THAT COMPLICATE DENTAL/DENTAL HYGIENE TREATMENT

Common Medical Conditions	Diseases That May Contraindicate Treatment	Diseases That Require Special Precautions	Diseases That May Endanger Health Professionals	Physiological States That Can Alter Treatment Procedures
Angina Pectoris	X	X		
Myocardial Infarction	X	X		
Congestive Heart Failure	X			
Asthma	X	X		
Chronic Bronchitis	X			
Liver Disease	X			
Diabetes	X	X		
Adrenal Insufficiency	X			
Hyperthyroidism	X			
Stroke	X			
Anemias	X			
Leukemia	X	X		
Hemophilia	X	X		
Radiation Therapy	X	X		
Rheumatic Heart Disease		X		
Congenital Cardiovascular Anomalies		X		
Hypertension		X		
Epilepsy		X		
Kidney Disorder		X		
Hepatitis B			X	
Tuberculosis			X	
Acquired Immunodeficiency Syndrome (AIDS)			X	
Pregnancy				X
Aging				X
Puberty				X

Table 2.4 • **NORMAL OR ACCEPTABLE FINDINGS FOR THE CLINICAL EXAMINATION**

Assessment Factor	Normal or Acceptable Findings
EXTRA ORAL EXAM	Straight gait, clear sclera, head and neck symmetrical, smooth and gliding TMJ, blood pressure range 100–140/60–90, pulse rate range 60–90, respirations 12–20 per min at rest, lymph nodes non-palpable.
INTRA ORAL EXAM	Smooth and shiny oral mucosa, rugae present, coral pink soft palate, tonsils (present or absent), tongue velvet texture on dorsal surface.
DENTAL EXAM	Occlusion class I, orthognathic profile, 28–32 teeth (full dentition), restorations well contoured to tooth structure, minimal areas of decay.
PERIODONTAL EXAM	Pink, knife-edged, flat, scalloped shaped gingival tissue, pocket probing depths 1 to 3 mm, loss of attachment ≤ to 3 mm, absence of bleeding and suppuration, minimal tooth mobility, furcation involvement limited, adequate attached gingiva (>1 mm).
ORAL HYGIENE EXAM	Plaque accumulation ≤ to 15 on the navy plaque index, minimal calculus (< 10 deposits), minimal stain (< 10 teeth containing stain).

dental exam, and the periodontal exam. It is not the intent of this book to provide a comprehensive review of the clinical examination; however, the pertinent components of each exam will be discussed. Table 2.4 lists the normal or acceptable findings associated with the clinical examination. Each of these procedures collects data through direct observation and examination; therefore, the information obtained is considered objective.

Observation is a skill that requires discipline and practice. It relies upon the conscious use of the senses: sight, smell, hearing, touch, taste. On the other hand, examination requires the development of such technical skills as palpation, tactile sensitivity, equipment usage, and instrumentation principles.

As previously mentioned, the assessment phase should be systematically organized to avoid errors; the same is true for each examination procedure. A specific routine or system should be established to direct the dental hygienist as the examination is performed. For instance, when conducting a periodontal probing evaluation, a suggested sequence would be to begin with the maxillary teeth (right quadrant facial aspect, left quadrant facial aspect, right quadrant lingual aspect, left quadrant lingual aspect) then proceed to the mandibular teeth (right quadrant facial aspect, left quadrant facial aspect, right quadrant lingual aspect, left quadrant lingual aspect).

Another example is the extra oral examination of the lymph nodes and temporomandibular joint (TMJ). A suggested systematic approach might be:

1. TMJ
2. Preauricular nodes
3. Postauricular nodes
4. Occipital nodes
5. Cervical chain
6. Supra clavicular nodes
7. Submaxillary or submandibular nodes
8. Submental nodes

EXTRA ORAL EXAM

The extra oral examination is conducted by observation and palpation of the exposed portions of the body. A general appraisal of the client's physical characteristics can be observed as the client is being escorted to the dental chair. Such details as gait, posture, speech patterns, obesity, and level of anxiety can give clues to the client's general state of health. In addition, specific observations of the head and neck areas should be made.

Eyes.   The eyes have been called the window to the soul and through the years have been examined to gain information about the client's overall physical condition. The following are some characteristics noted during evaluation of the eyes:

Reaction to light: The size of the pupil and its response to light can provide information about drug ingestion.

Eyelid shape: Drooping of the eyelid is a manifestation of Bell's palsy.

Color of the sclera: A yellowish tinge can indicate the presence of jaundice. If the sclera appears red, the client may be tired.

Skin and Lips.   The skin should be examined for any blemishes, moles, areas of pigmentation, open lesions, and/or swellings. Deviations from normal need to be described according to color, size, shape, location and whether the surface can be wiped away; for example, Ms. Jones has a pedunculated lesion approximately 2 mm in size, located 5 mm inferior to the ala of the nose. In addition, any irregularities in skin color, other than natural pigmentations, should be noted, such as pallor, cyanosis, or jaundice.

The lips are also inspected for the presence or absence of any abnormalities. The vermillion border should be easily traced as well as the commissures of the lips. Inflammation or ulceration can be the result of fungal or bacterial infection, vitamin deficiency, and habitual wetting.

Head and Neck.   The head and neck are observed for symmetry and examined by palpation for enlargement of the lymph nodes.

Temporomandibular Joint (TMJ).   Examination of the TMJ is performed to determine the presence or absence of soreness or asymmetry between the two sides. Bilateral palpation of the external surface of the joint during opening and closing of the mouth will determine the presence of crepitus, nonsymmetrical movement, and tenderness.

Vital Signs.   The vital signs taken by the dental hygienist during the extra oral examination include blood pressure, pulse, and respiration. These measurements are important when trying to screen clients for abnormal readings. However, it should be noted that higher readings are common in dental office settings because of the stressful situation perceived by the client. Therefore, screening will involve two or three evaluations during the course of the first appointment for accuracy.

   When determining the client's rate of respiration, the dental hygienist should take the measurement immediately following the pulse without informing the client. It has been documented that when the client is aware that his or her respiration is being monitored, he or she will unconsciously increase or decrease the amount of respirations during the given timeframe.

INTRA ORAL EXAMINATION

The intra oral examination has also been identified as the oral cancer examination and requires the skills of palpation and observation. When examining the intra oral areas a routine systematic procedure should be used and the following factors should be considered:

1. Color
2. Surface consistency or texture
3. Swelling or enlargement
4. Pain
5. Characteristics of lesion
6. Bleeding

Oral Mucosa.   The oral mucosa consists of the labial mucosa and the buccal mucosa. Inspection of this structure necessitates palpation and direct observation for deviations. Adequate light and the use of a mouth mirror or tongue blade to stretch the tissue facilitates this examination.

Hard Palate.   The hard palate is composed of keratinized tissue covering bony support. Examination findings might include a high vault, bony protuberance (tori palatinus), prominent rugae, or enlarged incisive papillae. The procedure to examine this structure is palpation and direct observation.

Soft Palate.   Notable findings of the soft palate include the presence or absence of swellings, petechiae, and unusual movement and/or size of the uvula. The soft palate cannot be palpated due to the gag reflex and is examined by visual observation only.

Oral Pharynx.   The oral pharynx should be inspected by depressing the posterior one-third of the tongue with a mouth mirror or tongue blade. The fauces and presence or absence of tonsils may be noted, as well as any abnormalities on the pharyngeal walls.

Tongue.   Examination of the tongue is performed by asking the client to extend his or her tongue and grasping it with a piece of gauze. The tongue is extended for evaluation of the dorsal surface and retracted from side to side for evaluation of the lateral borders. The ventral surface is inspected by asking the client to raise the tip of the tongue to the hard palate. Early signs of cancerous lesions and missing papillae are among some of the abnormal findings associated with the tongue.

DENTAL EXAMINATION

The examination of the teeth should be as systematic as the examination of the oral cavity. A sample examination procedure might include:

1. Count of the teeth
2. Identification of carious lesions
3. Identification of restorations (amount and type)
4. Defects in restorations
5. Fractures
6. Systemic effects (antibiotics, excessive fluoride)
7. Congenital defects (amelogenesis imperfecta, microdontia)
8. Occlusion

A complete and accurate dental examination and charting serves many purposes. It is used in treatment planning, forensic dentistry, and the correlation of radiographic findings. Treatment planning utilizes the examination to help prioritize treatment options. For example, a client presents with the need to replace a fixed bridge due to wear, and the periodontal examination reveals a periodontal condition. It would be wise to treat the periodontal condition first so that the foundation is strong enough to support the new bridge. In an example of forensic dentistry, the dental examination is helpful to identify individuals who are badly burned or decomposed to the point of being unrecognizable. The correlation of radiographic findings with the client's dental examination may assist the dental hygienist in distinguishing radiolucent restorative material from dental caries.

Occlusion.   The occlusal analysis is part of the dental examination and should consist of evaluation of all functional and parafunctional relationships. The possibility of trauma from occlusion should be identified, and the determination made as to whether it is primary or secondary occlusal trauma. In addition, the client's occlusion should be evaluated for fremitus, the presence of wear facets, deep vertical overbite, posterior bite collapse, horizontal overjet, and anterior open bite.

PERIODONTAL EXAMINATION

Performing the comprehensive periodontal examination is one of the most important functions of the dental hygienist. It is the basis for preventive and therapeutic treatment options that are well within our scope of practice. The periodontal examination is composed of nine clinical parameters that are used to assess periodontal disease:

1. Gingival assessment
2. Probing depth
3. Loss of attachment
4. Bleeding upon probing
5. Suppuration
6. Tooth mobility
7. Furcation involvement
8. Measurement of attached gingiva
9. Microbiological/host response monitoring.

Each of the parameters listed require both observation and examination of the structure under question.

Gingival Assessment.   The gingival tissues must be examined and findings recorded describing the color, size, contour, consistency, surface texture, and position. Specific attention should be given to the presence of recession and gingival clefts. Oral manifestations of gingival disorders such as herpetic gingivostomatitis or acute necrotizing ulcerative gingivitis should also be identified and recorded.

The examination procedure of the gingival tissues requires utilization of adequate lighting, a mouth mirror, and compressed air. The clinician needs a strong scientific knowledge base to be able to distinguish between normal and abnormal gingival conditions.

Probing Depth.   This measurement requires the use of a calibrated periodontal probe and a mouth mirror. Measurements are taken at six sites per tooth from the crest of the gingival margin to the epithelial attachment. These sites include the disto-buccal, direct buccal, mesio-buccal, disto-lingual, direct lingual, and mesio-lingual areas. The deepest reading at each site is recorded in the client's chart. Although this is one of the most commonly used clinical parameters in the assessment of periodontal disease, it should be noted that there are limitations associated with the accuracy of these measurements. Probing depth variations are dependent upon such limitations as the angulation of the probe, the force applied when probing, health of the tissue, diameter of the probe, difficulties with location and visibility of the probing site, and the presence of calculus deposits. These limitations can cause probing depth readings to vary as much as 1 mm to 2 mm.

Loss of Attachment.   The loss of attachment measurement identifies the true location of the epithelial junction by determining its distance from a fixed referenced
point on the tooth's surface. Probing depth determines the depth of the sulcular
crevice, but at times it does not represent the true clinical condition of the client.
For instance, if the gingival tissue is enlarged or receded, the measurements that
are made for probing depth do not identify when there is apical migration of the
junctional epithelium. Therefore, measurements associated with a fixed reference
point on the tooth's surface will be more accurate. The reference point can be the
margin of a crown, a restoration or the cemento-enamel junction (CEJ). Since the
probing depth measurement is usually taken first to calculate the loss of attachment of a given tooth, a more accurate reading is obtained by either adding or
subtracting the distance from the gingival margin to the fixed referenced point.

Bleeding on Probing.   Bleeding on probing is a clinical parameter used to identify
disease activity. Periodontal pocket depth measurements and loss of attachment
only provide information related to the history of a diseased condition. They do
not identify sites that are presently breaking down or undergoing active disease.
Therefore, the presence of bleeding is assessed.

There are two basic methods used to assess bleeding: bleeding on probing
(BOP) and bleeding on provocation. Each of these measurements is important
when trying to determine the client's disease status. Bleeding on probing measures the disease active at the base of the sulcus, which would be indicative of periodontitis. The probe is inserted into the sulcus and the presence or absence of
bleeding is recorded after 20 to 30 seconds. This type of bleeding evaluation can
be performed simultaneously with the measurement of pocket probing depth. The
second bleeding assessment method is bleeding on provocation. This method is
performed by inserting the probe 1 mm to 2 mm and sweeping it along the gingival margin. The bleeding that is elicited is indicative of gingivitis.

Some researchers believe that bleeding on probing or provocation is a valid
predictor of disease activity when demonstrating health (no bleeding present).
However, to state that active disease is present when bleeding is noted, then the
limitations previously mentioned associated with probing need to be identified
and evaluated. For example, was the probing force too great? or was the probe
incorrectly adapted? In clinical practice we are not as critical as we are in research
when it comes to false positive readings because the client's overall condition is
usually evaluated on more than one site.

Suppuration.   The presence or absence of suppuration is another clinical parameter that is used to identify disease activity. However, this parameter is considered a
definite marker of inflammation. It is identified during the probing depth evaluation as a purulent exudate. In extremely active diseased sites this exudate might be
spontaneously expelled from the gingival sulcus.

Tooth Mobility.   Identification of tooth mobility is part of the periodontal examination. It is performed with the end of two instrument handles. One handle end is
placed on the buccal aspect and one on the lingual aspect of the tooth. The tooth
is then gently pushed back and forth. The direction and degree of tooth mobility

is classified and recorded on the client's chart to help determine the prognosis of the tooth.

Furcation Involvement. Furcation involvement refers to the detection of missing bone between the roots of teeth. It is best identified with the use of a Naber's probe. This probe is designed specifically to measure bone loss between tooth roots. Furcation involvement is classified according to its degree of involvement and recorded in the client's chart.

Measure Attached Gingiva. We discussed the measurement of the loss of attachment, which is related to the location of the junctional epithelium. The measurement of the attached gingiva is associated with the keratinized portion of the gingiva that is firmly attached to the bone. This measurement is performed with the use of a standard probe placed on the outside of the tissue. A measurement is made from the gingival margin to the mucogingival junction. The pocket probing depth measurement is subtracted from this measurement and the amount of attached gingiva remaining is identified.

Microbiological and Host Response Testing. Microbiological and host response testing is a fairly new clinical parameter used to assess the level of disease activity. These tests were developed because periodontal disease is multifactorial. Different types of bacteria have been found to produce different types of periodontal disease; the way in which the body responds to the infection will ultimately determine the level of breakdown (see Table 2.5) The tests that have been developed include DNA probing, bacteriological culturing, sulcular temperature evaluation, and host response enzyme identification systems. During periodontal assessment these tests will provide pertinent information concerning the client's disease status, as specific as an individual site or as general as an overall interpretation.

ORAL HYGIENE

The oral hygiene evaluation can be performed at any point in the assessment process, but is most relevant when related to the periodontal evaluation. At this point during assessment, the dental hygienist has a good indication of the level of disease present in the client's mouth. There are three factors to be considered in the oral hygiene evaluation and all have significance to periodontal and dental health.

The first is *bacterial plaque.* Bacterial plaque has been identified as the primary

Table 2.5 • **DISEASE ACTIVITY FACTORS**

Pathogens		Host Resistance		Disease Status
	⟶		=	
Low Level	⟶	High Level	=	Health
Low Level	⟶	Low Level	=	Stable or Active Disease
High Level	⟶	Low Level	=	Active Disease
High Level	⟶	High Level	=	Stable

etiological agent in both caries and periodontal disease. It is evaluated by the clinician with the use of plaque indices that identify the amount and distribution of the plaque on the tooth surface. The data collected can be calculated into mean plaque scores for the entire dentition or separated into individual site scores. Since this is directly related to the client's home care regimen, the client should be an active participant during the discovery and measurement of the plaque.

The second factor associated with the oral hygiene examination is *dental calculus*. Although dental calculus is not considered an etiological agent in periodontal disease, its presence can affect the formation and propagation of bacterial plaque. Therefore, the location and amount of calculus present on the tooth surface should be noted and recorded in the client's chart.

Stain is the last factor evaluated during the oral hygiene examination. This factor has no true clinical significance but can cause considerable concern to the client. Stains can arise from any number of sources and are classified by formation (exogenous or endogenous) and by location (intrinsic or extrinsic). Documentation of dental stain is necessary during the assessment phase, since removal of heavy stain requires a considerable amount of time and effort. The identification of this condition is important so that the appropriate amount of time can be allocated during treatment planning.

RADIOGRAPHIC EXAMINATION

It is beyond the scope of this book to focus in detail on the interpretation and diagnosis of dental radiographs, but some general observations and guidelines can be presented concerning the role of the radiographic survey in the assessment phase of care. According to FDA guidelines, radiographs should be taken based on diagnostic need rather than on any standing routine (Health Science Division of Eastman Kodak, 1988). However, since attempts to identify specific criteria that will accurately predict a high probability of finding carious lesions have not been successful, a time-based schedule for taking radiographs was recommended by the panel established by the Health Science Division of Eastman Kodak Company (1988). The schedule provides a range of recommended exposure intervals derived from the results of numerous clinical research studies. Each schedule interval categorizes clients by type of visit—new or maintenance.

The schedule guidelines recommended that radiographs should be taken on the child client prior to eruption of the first permanent tooth and then again at a point during the transitional dentition. If the child is a new client with a full primary dentition and proximal surfaces of primary teeth that cannot be visualized or probed, a posterior bitewing examination is also suggested. During the transitional dentition period, the new child client should have an individualized radiographic examination consisting of periapical/occlusal radiographs and posterior bitewings, or a panoramic examination and posterior bitewings. For maintenance visits, a posterior bitewing exam at six-month intervals is recommended if the client demonstrates a high risk for caries. If caries activity is low, then a posterior bitewing exam should only be performed at twelve- to twenty-four-month intervals.

The adolescent client is classified as having a permanent dentition prior to eruption of third molars. As a new client, the individualized radiographic examination should consist of posterior bitewings and selected periapicals. A full-mouth intra oral examination is appropriate when the client presents with clinical evidence of generalized dental disease or a history of extensive dental treatment. Posterior bitewing examination is recommended for maintenance visits at six- to twelve-month intervals if the client is at risk for disease, and eighteen- to thirty-six-month intervals if risk factors are low. Assessment of growth and development, especially of the developing third molars, requires a periapical or panoramic examination.

Recommendations by the panel for the adult client are identical to the adolescent client, except for maintenance intervals. The adult client who is at risk for caries should have a posterior bitewing examination performed at twelve- to eighteen-month intervals, and twenty-four- to thirty-six-month intervals when at low risk.

All clients should be evaluated for periodontal disease. Individualized radiographic examinations consisting of selected periapical and/or bitewing radiographs should be taken for areas where periodontal disease can be demonstrated clinically. Emergency radiographs are taken to provide sufficient information for an immediate diagnosis of an acute condition. These can be limited to one periapical film or may include several films, depending on the area involved.

LABORATORY TESTS

Laboratory tests should be employed whenever possible to clarify assessment findings and provide additional information. In dentistry and dental hygiene, there are a number of laboratory tests that can be utilized. They include, but are not limited to, the following:

1. Biopsy or cytology of suspicious oral lesions: Most pathology labs will provide the materials necessary to take a sample specimen without causing alarm to the client.

2. Bacteriological cultures: As previously mentioned, bacteriological cultures can provide information related to the type of pathogen involved in a periodontal condition. These cultures can also be combined with antibiotic sensitivity testing to aid in the identification of appropriate treatment options.

3. DNA probes, specifically the DMDX test or the Pathotec test (Biotechnica, Inc.): These are laboratory tests which evaluate the DNA of the plaque sample and determine the level of pathogenic microorganisms. Reports take approximately ten days and classify the presence of the pathogen as low, moderate, or high.

4. Phase contrast microscopy: Although the scientific value of this test is questionable, it can be used as a motivational tool to reinforce home care regimens. Many clients are unaware that the plaque in their mouths is alive and the organisms are motile. Research has determined that the level of mobility of the microorganisms in plaque can be correlated to the degree of maturity.

5. Host response tests: These tests, as mentioned earlier, are used to assess the client's present disease status. Most are performed by taking a sample of the client's gingival crevicular fluid (GCF) and analyzing its contents for enzymes that are indicative of active disease. Some of the enzymes that are analyzed

include: aspartate aminotransferase (AST), elastase, B-glucuronidase (BG), and collagenase.

6. Modified Snyder test: This laboratory test is available to provide information relating to the presence of acid-producing organisms in the saliva. The information generated from this test correlates well to decay rates and can identify clients who are susceptible to caries.

CLINICAL PHOTOGRAPHY

The value of clinical photography is for the documentation of assessment findings. It is also helpful to evaluate and compare post treatment results. Suggested photographs for a general assessment include five views:

1. Anterior view of the maxillary and mandibular teeth in occlusion

2. Right buccal view of the teeth in occlusion

3. Left buccal view of the teeth in occlusion

4. Occlusal view of maxillary teeth and palate

5. Occlusal view of the mandibular teeth and floor of the mouth

Specific oral conditions can also be photographed to provide closeup views of a single tooth or gingival area. Clinical photography is used most often as a means of documentation for legal purposes and case studies.

DOCUMENTATION

The second component of the assessment phase is documentation of the database. Although the following discussion of documentation is directed toward the recording of data accumulated during the assessment phase, documentation is integral to all phases of the dental hygiene process of care.

Documentation of the data that has been collected is essential for making a diagnosis and developing a treatment plan. The written dental hygiene record enables the dental hygienist to review all pertinent information with the dentist to devise a treatment plan ensuring that all problems identified in the examination and discovered upon integration of findings are addressed. In addition, accurately documented baseline findings form the standard for comparison of subsequent data collection, allowing the dental hygienist to validate, clarify, or update preliminary diagnoses. The goal is to ensure the provision of consistent individualized care.

The dental hygiene record is also a legal document. The relationship that exists between the health care provider and the client is in most cases a legal contract. It may be used to evaluate liability in a malpractice litigation, document client compliance, determine the extent of injury in compensation claims, and/or substantiate specific treatment modalities for reimbursement. Therefore, it is important that the information listed in the dental record be accurate, legible, complete, and comprehensive. The information recorded as part of the assessment phase may protect the client, the care providers, and the employer when situations arise.

Lastly, documentation provides the foundation for dental hygiene research. The information found in the dental hygiene record may be utilized as a source for identification of research topics specific to dental hygiene practice. Validation of dental hygiene diagnoses, comparison of client responses to dental hygiene interventions, and development of dental hygienist/client relationships are potential areas of exploration. The accumulation of a body of knowledge has been identified by the ADHA as a way to define dental hygiene as a profession and refine the dental hygiene process of care.

Criteria for Dental Hygiene Records

The criteria for dental hygiene records cannot be emphasized enough because of their role in diagnosis, treatment planning, treatment itself, and legal ramifications. The following criteria can be established as a strict set of criteria for all dental records. All records should be:

ACCURATE

The need for accuracy in dental hygiene records is fairly obvious. For example, if the wrong tooth is marked for extraction, the results can be disastrous. Such details as the spelling of a client's name or a correct, current address can prevent gross errors or in the least, embarrassment. Inaccuracies or omissions in dental records tend to cast doubt on the entire record and on the integrity of the treatment. In dental hygiene specifically, accurate chartings of periodontal information is mandatory for treatment to be successful.

LEGIBLE

To be of any use, the dental record must be readable, not only to the dental hygienist, but to anyone who might need the information in the record, such as a receptionist, dentist, another hygienist, or even an attorney. Therefore, record entries should be made in black ink (unless visual chartings require colored pencil), and the record should be protected against smudges and/or water spots.

COMPLETE AND COMPREHENSIVE

The complete and comprehensive dental hygiene record should contain a clear and concise recording of all essential information. Any record system has certain essential components, and the dental hygiene record is not considered complete unless it includes the following:

1. Business information, including the client's name, address, phone number, physicians name, and all other pertinent personal data. It is obvious that the dental hygienist must know who he or she is treating and record that information.

2. Client history, both medical and dental. This history should describe present and past conditions that may have contraindications for or complicate treatment.

3. Consent forms, always signed prior to any type of treatment or evaluation procedure. The consent provides legal documentation for the health care provider to proceed. It is a statement signed by the client stating that he or she is consenting to the examination. After the examination is performed and a treatment plan developed, the client should be asked to sign either a contract or an additional consent form. This additional consent indicates that the client is willing to proceed with treatment.

4. Intra and extra oral examinations.

5. Dental chart, including provision for charting existing conditions, restorations, missing teeth, clinical and radiographic findings, and occlusion.

6. Periodontal examination record, including periodontal charting and the gingival assessment.

7. Oral hygiene record, consisting of plaque, calculus, and gingival indices.

8. Written treatment plan, including treatment options, treatment dates, client's acceptance or rejection, modifications, or changes made during the actual course of treatment.

9. Dental radiographs, identified with the client's name and date the radiographs were taken.

10. Treatment rendered, including any and all treatment performed, fees charged, or conversations with client regarding same, dated and initialed by the provider of care.

One issue that comes to mind when discussing the dental record is infection control, specifically cross contamination. It is very easy for the clinician to contaminate the dental hygiene records when recording information. The forms within the dental chart are handled during the examination with hands that have touched the client and are considered infectious. One method of charting that helps to control potential cross contamination is the use of a clear plastic shield. The shield is placed on top of dental record forms and moved down the forms as the clinician records the information. This method does not eliminate the potential for cross contamination, but does help to minimize it.

However, there are two methods that can be used to eliminate record cross contamination. The first is having a dental assistant, who records assessment findings as the exam is being performed. This is effective, but costly, because two people are needed to perform the same procedure. The second is the use of computers. Today there are many dental charting systems available to assist the dental hygienist in collecting assessment data. These systems record the information on a computer disk, and standard forms can then be printed out for the client's chart. These forms are typically very graphic and easy to read—a plus for submission to insurance companies. Voice Victor™ is a computer system developed by Prodentec Inc. utilizing voice activation. The dental hygienist simply talks into a headset while performing the assessment procedures and data is entered directly into the computer. Although these systems save time and reduce the possibility of cross contamination, they are considered expensive.

Summary

The assessment phase of the dental hygiene process of care consists of the accumulation and documentation of information about a client. Data collection involves interviewing, observation, and physical examination, and concludes with documentation of the information in the client's medical record. Assessment involves interaction between the dental hygienist and the client, and requires a broad knowledge base as well as specific interpersonal and technical skills. Assessment is a continuous activity that begins at the time of the initial appointment and continues throughout all additional appointments. It forms the foundation for subsequent phases of the dental hygiene process of care—diagnosis, planning, implementation, and evaluation.

REFERENCES

Bellack, J., & Bamford, P. (1984). *Nursing assessment.* Belmont, California: Wadsworth.

Benicewicz, D., & Metzger, C. (1989). Supervision and practice of dental hygienists: Report of ADHA survey. *Journal of Dental Hygiene, 63,* 173–180.

Boyer, E., & Gupta, G. (1990). Dentist involvement in care provided by the dental hygienist. *Journal of Dental Hygiene, 64,* 273–277.

Brady, W., & Martinoff, J. (1980). Validity of health history data collected from dental patients and patients' perceptions of health status. *Journal of the American Dental Association, 101,* 642–645.

Chamber, D., & Abrams, R. (1986). *Dental communication* (p. 77). Norwalk, Connecticut: Appleton-Century-Crofts.

Enelow, A., & Swisher, S. (1979). *Interviewing and patient care* (2nd ed., pp. 40–41). New York: Oxford University Press.

Fenlon, M., & McCartlan, B. (1992). Validity of patient self completed health questionnaire in a primary care dental practice. *Community Dental Oral Epidemiology, 20,*130–132.

Health Science Division of Eastman Kodak Company. (1988). *Guidelines for prescribing dental radiographs.* Rochester, NY: Author.

Ingersol, B. (1982). *Behavioral aspects in dentistry.* New York: Appleton-Century-Crofts.

Slots, J. (1986). Bacterial specificity in adult periodontitis: A summary of recent work. *Journal of Clinical Periodontology, 13,* 912–917.

Theilade, E. (1986). The non-specific theory in microbial etiology of inflammatory periodontal disease. *Journal of Clinical Periodontology, 13,* 905–911.

Exercise 2.1   Types of Data

The following is a list of data. Indicate whether each item is subjective or objective by placing an (X) in the appropriate column.

Data	Subjective	Objective
1. Gait is staggered		
2. Blood pressure is 180/95		
3. "My tooth hurts"		
4. "My gums are tender"		
5. Periodontal pocket readings 3 mm		
6. Seems nervous		
7. Tooth #8 is fractured		
8. Generalized decalcification		
9. "I need anesthesia"		
10. Class III occlusion		

Identify each of the following as historical or current.

Data	Historical	Current
11. No prior dental treatment		
12. Brushes twice daily		
13. "I used to floss"		
14. "I'm allergic to penicillin"		
15. "When I brush my gums bleed"		
16. Two epileptic seizures last month		
17. "I had braces"		
18. "My teeth were bleached"		
19. "The light is in my eyes"		
20. Controlled diabetic		

Exercise 2.2 Assessment Sequence

Arrange the following assessment activities in the correct sequence of performance.

_____ Client Consent

_____ Medical History

_____ Extra Oral Exam

_____ Pathogen Tests

_____ Gingival Assessment

Exercise 2.3 Identification of Medical History Conditions

The first phase of the assessment process is the review of the medical-dental history and physical assessment of vital signs. Using the chart below fill in the correct information in each column.

Finding	Risk Factor	Medical Clearance or Premedication	Continue Comprehensive Charting
Example: Client reports mitral valve prolapse	Subacute bacterial endocarditis	Yes	No
Diabetes			
Hypotension			
Pregnancy			

CHAPTER 3

Dental Hygiene Diagnosis

Learning Outcomes

At the completion of the chapter the reader should be able to:

1. Describe the significance of developing a dental hygiene diagnosis in the dental hygiene process of care

2. Differentiate between a dental and dental hygiene diagnosis

3. Categorize data to aid in the formulation of the diagnostic statement

4. Formulate a dental hygiene diagnosis based upon a list of assessment findings

5. Analyze assessment findings and critically evaluate the significance

INTRODUCTION

A diagnosis is essentially a statement that identifies the existence of a condition from its signs and symptoms. This definition applies whether the diagnostician is a health care provider, lawyer, electrician, or mechanic. The subject matter of the diagnosis consists of those areas in which the diagnostician possesses a level of expertise. For example, lawyers write diagnoses pertaining to elements of law, electricians identify electrical system malfunctions, and auto mechanics diagnose problems pertaining to the accurate servicing of vehicles. Dental hygienists are responsible for health promotion, disease prevention, and oral health maintenance to prevent the occurrence or recurrence of oral disease.

The dental hygiene diagnosis has been defined as a formal statement of the dental hygienist's decision regarding the actual or potential problems of a client that are amenable to treatment through the dental hygiene process of care (Darby, 1990). It identifies the scope of dental hygiene practice by clarifying the role of the dental hygienist and defining dental hygiene's unique contribution to oral health care. In addition, the dental hygiene diagnosis forms the basis of dental hygiene education and creates a sense of direction for research and future trends. However, the most important benefit of the dental hygiene diagnosis is to facilitate individualized care planning.

In general, a diagnosis is comprised of the following (Taylor, Lillie, and Lemone, 1993):

1. A short concise two-part statement of a problem and possible etiology

2. A statement of a conclusion resulting from identification of a pattern or relationship between signs and symptoms

3. A basis of subjective and objective data

4. Reference to a condition that the diagnostician is licensed to treat

5. Validation with the client whenever possible

DEVELOPING THE DENTAL HYGIENE DIAGNOSIS

Many models have been developed for diagnostic decision making. All models analyze and synthesize data collected during assessment through deductive reasoning and determine a diagnosis. As with any decision-making process, many factors need to be considered. The diagnostician must process the information and make judgments based on clinical reasoning and problem-solving skills. The nursing model of diagnosis (Gordon, 1987) broadens the already established medical and dental models to include the health functioning of individuals. It describes the actual or potential health problems that nurses are able to treat. The following steps in the development of a diagnosis are based on the nursing model and form the basis for independent decision making with a focus on client problems requiring treatment within the dental hygiene process of care. Specifically, the two steps involved in the development of a diagnosis include *data processing* and *diagnosis formulation*. The end product is a concise statement that identifies the client's problem and possible etiology (Figure 3.1). The dental hygiene diagnostic statement forms the foundation from which the plan of care is designed, implemented, and evaluated.

DATA PROCESSING

The information collected during the assessment phase must be processed before it can be utilized to develop a diagnosis and care plan. We all use data processing, the intellectual thought process, every day to determine the existence of a problem and its possible etiology.

Dental hygienists and other health care professionals use critical thinking skills to assist in the processing of data, to collect and interpret information, and to make sound judgments that contribute to good decisions. While the level of decision making may vary, data processing is based on critical thinking.

There are many characteristics associated with critical thinking: The critical thinker uses a rational, fair, purposeful, and goal-directed thought process. The

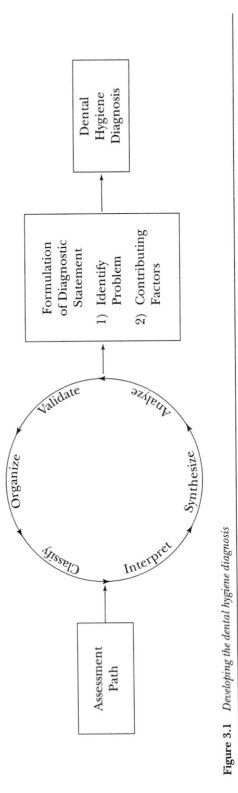

Figure 3.1 *Developing the dental hygiene diagnosis*

following statements identify some specific characteristics of a critical thinker (Paul, 1988).

1. Explores the thinking that underlies emotions and feelings.
2. Suspends judgments when there is a lack of sufficient evidence.
3. Develops criteria for evaluation and applies them fairly and accurately.
4. Evaluates the credibility of sources used to justify beliefs.
5. Makes interdisciplinary connections and uses insights from one subject to illuminate and correct other subjects.
6. Distinguishes facts from ideals.
7. Examines assumptions that underlie thoughts and behaviors.
8. Makes plausible inferences and conclusions.
9. Distinguishes the relevant from the irrelevant and the important from the trivial.
10. Seeks out evidence and gives evidence when questioned.

Finding patterns and relationships and making sound inferences are critical thinking skills used in developing a dental hygiene diagnosis. Although data processing will be discussed as the first step in diagnosis, it is not completely isolated. These events are active rather than static and occur continuously throughout the dental hygiene process of care. Data processing includes the classification, interpretation, and validation of information collected during the assessment phase.

Classification

During the assessment of a client, the dental hygienist accumulates a massive volume of data that may be difficult to manage in total. However, by organizing and classifying the data into more manageable categories, the information may not seem so overwhelming. This type of information classification also stimulates discrimination between data and allows the dental hygienist to focus on data that are pertinent to the client's needs.

Classification involves the sorting of information into specific categories. Frequently this process is facilitated by the framework established in the assessment phase (see Table 3.1). As information is classified, it becomes clear how diagnostic statements can develop within one category or between two or more categories (see Table 3.2).

Table 3.1 • **ASSESSMENT CATEGORIES**

Chief Complaint	Hard Tissue
General Systemic	Soft Tissue
Dental History	Periodontal
Oral Habit	Oral Hygiene
Nutrition	Radiographic Survey

Table 3.2 • **DATA CLASSIFICATION**

Data	Assessment Category Classification
Myocardial infarction	General Systemic
Flosses daily	Oral Hygiene
Generalized recession	Periodontal
Pain on right side	Chief Complaint
Bleeding on probing	Periodontal
Ulceration in mucobuccal fold	Soft Tissue
10 restorations	Dental History
Cheek biting	Oral Habit

Categorization also assists the dental hygienist to begin to identify and collect missing data during the assessment phase. For example, the client states that his gums used to bleed and that he would seek regular dental hygiene treatment approximately every three months. Classification of this information reveals a missing component—current status of gingival health. Therefore, the dental hygienist might (1) question the client regarding the present status of his gingival tissue (Do you still have bleeding gums?), and (2) determine if the client is still maintaining frequent dental hygiene treatment (When was the last time you had dental hygiene treatment?). Although some of this information will be gathered during the intra oral examination, it is important to make the client a participant and determine his level of awareness.

Interpretation

The second step in the processing of data is interpretation. What does the data mean? Data interpretation relies upon the critical thinking skills of the dental hygienist and includes the cognitive processes of analysis, synthesis, inductive reasoning, and deductive reasoning. Analysis of the database is used to examine each piece of information, identify deviations from normal, and identify patterns or relationships in the data. Synthesis means combining parts or elements to generate explanations of the symptoms. Inductive reasoning is used to find possible patterns in information and extend them to predict new information. Lastly, deductive reasoning begins with a generalization and proceeds to discover specific facts. In general, data interpretation is necessary to identify significant data, compare with standards or norms, recognize deviations, describe abnormalities, and analyze the abnormalities with respect to significance.

Identification of significant data requires that the dental hygienist have a good grasp of the clinical normal, both from textbook courses and from observation of many "normal" clients. The term normal is used here to distinguish the conditions that are usually present in the oral cavity and represent the clinical picture of health. Some clinicians use the terms "within normal limits" (WLN) as a modifier to describe insignificant findings.

Recognizing deviations from the norm requires that the dental hygienist be on guard. Being able to recite the definition of normal for any given factor or condition is of little value if the hygienist does not recognize abnormal findings when they appear.

Describing the abnormality or deviation from normal assists the dental hygienist when formulating a written diagnosis. This description should be accurate and concise. For example, the term periodontitis would not greatly aid us in selecting an appropriate course of treatment. However, a brief description of major findings would be more likely to direct the plan of care:

> 5-7 mm periodontal pockets in all posterior sextants, suppuration is present in the maxillary right and mandibular left posterior sextants, DNA probe analysis reveals a high level of pathogens in all posterior sextants, plaque scores identify interproximal neglect.

Although this is time-consuming, the description tells us precisely what is happening and strongly suggests an etiologic factor to be investigated. It helps the dental hygienist individualize care. In this respect, a description is more valuable than a single term that can be misleading.

Analyzing the abnormality or data collected requires the dental hygienist to determine if the finding is significant but not critical, potentially serious, or absolutely critical to the oral health (or systemic health) of the client. Judgment should be withheld as to the exact nature, significance, and scientific name of the findings in question, but possibilities should be considered, of both the nature of the abnormality and its etiology.

The step of data interpretation is applied throughout the assessment phase or immediately following the assessment phase. As previously mentioned, the abnormal observations are classified or grouped into the assessment categories such as general systemic, soft tissue, periodontal, dental, or oral hygiene.

The following is a brief discussion of some typical classifications and interpretations of data collected during the assessment phase.

GENERAL SYSTEMIC CATEGORY

From the general appraisal and medical history of the client, a sketch of the overall condition can be made. This sketch should include any finding that may have significance in dental or oral conditions, or in dental hygiene treatment. The following are some examples.

1. Normal, healthy, 30-year-old woman with an allergy to penicillin and gastric intolerance to aspirin.

2. 18-year-old man, diabetic on daily injectable insulin. He is rather obese; his diet is not well controlled. He seems apathetic and displays difficulty in communication.

3. Normal, healthy, 82-year-old woman with a history of arthritis that is fairly well controlled by two aspirin daily. Blood pressure is 180/100, which is within normal limits for her age.

These examples summarize and highlight the comprehensive medical and general appraisal of the clients and should capsulize those findings likely to be significant in dental/dental hygiene treatment. In many cases, the general systemic findings may contain nothing that is significant to us and will therefore not be a factor in developing the diagnosis. In other cases, the complexity and severity of a client's systemic problem may preclude dental/dental hygiene treatment at this time. However, in most cases, the general systemic findings will influence the dental situation in one of three ways.

The first is indirect influence. Findings that require precaution or premedication, but may not directly affect the disease or treatment, exert indirect influence on the situation. For example, a history of rheumatic fever requiring prophylactic antibiotics, or an allergy to a commonly used anesthetic are considered indirect influences.

Data from the general systemic findings can also exert a direct influence on dental/dental hygiene treatment. For example, diabetes may affect the severity of periodontal disease and loss of salivary flow may predispose the client directly to caries. Less obvious, severe arthritis may prevent plaque control, thereby aggravating most oral diseases.

Lastly, reverse influence is used to describe situations that are present due to dental or dental hygiene disorders. An example would be headaches and earaches related to occlusal or TMJ disorders. Sore throats may be secondary to pericoronitis of a partially impacted third molar.

The extent to which a systemic finding will influence treatment often depends on what type of treatment is contemplated. Bleeding disorders or hemophilia of various types may not be significant if treatment is to consist of placing dental sealants, or providing fluoride therapy, but it would be absolutely critical if subgingival scalings were indicated. Since we probably will not establish a treatment plan until the client's complete diagnosis is developed, the systemic findings that we note would include any or all that may potentially influence treatment.

SOFT TISSUE CATEGORY

Following the examination of the external head and neck, lymph-node palpation, and the intra oral soft tissue (oral cancer) examination, any significant findings can be listed briefly. Typically these would include, but are not limited to, lesions, swellings or nodules, asymmetry, abnormal color or surface texture, or pain or tenderness on palpation.

If the findings and their history are readily explainable, such as an ulcerated palatal lesion that the client says is a result of hot pizza, it may be considered insignificant. Findings that are significant because of their clinical appearance and history, such as a unilateral swelling of the floor of the mouth which the client states comes and goes, should be briefly summarized. The following are examples of common soft-tissue descriptions:

1. Small (5 mm diameter), fibrous nodule on the right buccal mucosa near commissure; client reports occasionally biting, probable fibroma.

2. Multiple petechiae spread over soft palate causing no pain or tenderness; client unaware of presence.

3. Small (2 mm diameter), painless, indurated ulcer on left lateral border of tongue; client unaware of presence.

4. Swelling and tenderness in right submandibular lymph node of recent onset. It is probably associated with a decayed tooth in the right mandibular molar region.

From the history and clinical picture, the soft-tissue abnormality may be ignored, evaluated more thoroughly with a biopsy, or monitored and reevaluated at another interval. Keep in mind that the abnormality may be related to other aspects of the findings or to other factors.

PERIODONTAL CATEGORY

It is advisable in the periodontal category to be very specific in terminology in order to describe exactly the periodontal situation present. For example, the term "gingivitis" has a very definite meaning, especially as differentiated from "periodontitis." The former refers to an inflammatory condition involving soft tissues of the periodontium, but not the alveolar bone. The latter refers to a disease state that has resulted in destruction and loss of alveolar bone as determined through observation (probing) and radiographic evidence. These specific terms and others like them (e.g., juvenile periodontitis) can be modified to further refine the diagnosis. A periodontal condition can be acute or chronic in nature, localized or generalized in distribution, mild or severe in its apparent rate of progression or advanced in its apparent state of progression. These are but a few of the modifiers that can be applied to a periodontal condition. The following examples illustrate the periodontal description.

1. Normal, healthy periodontium with local areas of recession maxillary molars, and mandibular canines.
2. Acute gingivitis, generalized, with bleeding and hypertrophic tissue interproximally. 3 to 5 mm pockets posterior.
3. Chronic advanced severe periodontitis, generalized with 50 percent or more bone loss, and class III mobility throughout.
4. Periodontitis, generally incipient with localized severe lesions (5 to 8 mm) pockets between #2 and #3, and furcation involvement #15 and #30.
5. Chronic periodontitis, mild for age (70 years) less than 15 percent bone loss, slight mobility of lower anteriors.
6. Acute necrotizing ulcerative gingivitis with loss of papillae, marked halitosis and severe discomfort.

The careful and exhaustive periodontal assessment evaluation makes the interpretation and description of the client's condition clear. This concise synopsis of the client's condition helps to formulate specific diagnostic statements.

ORAL HYGIENE CATEGORY

The client's oral hygiene status is directly related to the etiology and treatment of the periodontal condition as well as other oral conditions. Taking into account the levels of plaque, calculus, and stain observed on the teeth we can roughly generalize the client's oral hygiene practices. To provide some objectivity during the assessment phase, criteria-based indices should be used to determine the amount of plaque, calculus, and stain present (see Chapter 2). The following are some examples of the oral hygiene description.

1. Heavy plaque accumulation present on the buccal aspect of the posterior teeth. Moderate supra and sub gingival calculus accumulation present on the buccal aspect of the maxillary first molars and the lingual of the mandibular incisors. Gingivitis index score of 2.5 using the Loe and Silness gingival index. Client states once daily brushing in AM.

2. Moderate plaque accumulation on the interproximal surfaces of all teeth. Light calculus accumulation present subgingivally in the molar areas. Interproximal bleeding present upon probing. Client states brushing three times daily but no flossing.

3. Light plaque accumulation present at the gingival margins of all teeth. No calculus accumulation. Client states twice daily brushing and once daily flossing.

DENTAL CATEGORY

The dental description involves the data that is collected during the resortative charting procedure. This information relates to the presence of caries, malformations, occlusal wear, abrasion, erosion, intrinsic stain, and defective (faulty) restoration.

Caries is the most common dental disease and is produced by bacterial plaque. The contributing factors include the type, and intake frequency of carbohydrate substrates.

Malformations that are dysfunctional include the following characteristics: enamel defects, poorly formed or "chalky" that do not provide the structural strength; abnormal crown morphology that does not provide function and occlusal support or has severe anatomic anomalies (accessory cusps, deep developmental grooves); poorly formed teeth that may have mild problems that should be watched; or severe problems that may jeopardize the tooth. Nevertheless, the effects of malformation must be considered in the dental diagnosis.

Occlusal wear represents a form of dysfunction based on the nature and severity of the wear in relation to the age of the client. Types of wear patterns to consider include the following:

1. Faceting, wear spots in the enamel involving few teeth, may be from an adjustment to occlusion changes or indicative of occlusal trauma, which can produce mobility, tenderness, and severe localized bony defects in the presence of periodontal inflammation.

2. Faceting on all teeth in both arches may also be from an occlusion adjustment or it may indicate a bruxing or clenching habit that can lead to serious periodontal damage.

Abrasion and *erosion* can cause severe loss of tooth structure. Abrasion produced by mechanical means is considered to be severe wear of the enamel or cementum.

Once the enamel or cementum is lost, the exposed dentin is highly sensitive and susceptible to further attrition. Toothbrushing is the most common etiologic factor—stiff bristle brushes usually are considered the primary culprits when used in a back-and-forth brushing technique. Even soft nylon brushes can aggravate existing abrasions if used in a sawing motion, since the V-groove most often created at the gingiva of the tooth directs the bristles into the same pattern that originally produced the abrasion.

This situation makes effective plaque control difficult and leads to further abrasion and gingival tissue damage. Some abraded areas can be carefully maintained with a soft toothbrush and a non-abrasive brushing technique. Desensitization of the abraded area can help reduce discomfort.

Erosion is generally considered to be a chemically induced loss of tooth structure that is often related to unusual dietary patterns such as lemon sucking and self-induced vomiting as seen with bulimia. The presence of citrus fruits and other highly acidic foods in the mouth seldom results in loss of tooth structure by itself, so erosion is generally seen and treated in combination with mechanical abrasion.

Validation

Validation is the third step in data processing, following classification and interpretation. It is an attempt to verify the accuracy of data interpretation. This may be accomplished by direct interaction with the client or significant other(s), consultation with other health care professionals, or comparison of data with an authoritative reference.

Validation is an important component of the diagnostic process. It assists the dental hygienist in recognizing errors, isolating discrepancies, and identifying the need for additional information. There is always some risk that the hygienist's interpretation is less than accurate. Therefore, it is important to remain open to change as new data and insights are presented.

FORMULATION OF DENTAL HYGIENE DIAGNOSIS

Following data processing, the dental hygiene diagnostic statement is formulated. The diagnostic statement focuses on the client's individual needs. It determines the potential or actual problems that can be prevented, minimized or resolved by the dental hygienist through independent or interdependent interventions. The diagnostic statement becomes the framework for the subsequent phases of planning, implementation, and evaluation.

Components of the Diagnostic Statement

The dental hygiene diagnostic statement consists of two parts joined by the phrase "related to." In writing dental hygiene diagnoses, the dental hygienist should remember that the diagnostic statement contains two parts. The first part is a determination of the client's condition or problem; the second part identifies the contributing factors (Taptich, Iyer, & Bernocchi-Losey, 1989).

The client's condition is stated according to the data processed during the assessment phase. It also describes to what degree the condition is present. Qualifying phrases precede or follow the condition statement to identify stages or levels. For example, the term "potential" means that the individual is at risk for a problem. This qualifier can be used to describe a dental hygiene diagnosis such as "potential for bone loss." Another qualifier is the term "possible," which means that the condition may be present, but more data needs to be collected and validated. The dental hygienist writes a diagnosis of "possible dexterity difficulties." Table 3.3 lists some additional qualifiers and examples for use.

The etiology constitutes the second part of the dental hygiene diagnosis. To prevent, minimize, or alleviate the condition, the dental hygienist must know why it is occurring. The etiology reflects the environmental, psychological, sociocultural, and physiological factors believed to be related or contributing to the health

Table 3.3 • DIAGNOSTIC QUALIFIERS

Qualifier	Definition	Diagnostic Example
Acute	Severe, rapid onset, of short duration	Acute dentinal pain
Altered	A change from the usual	Altered emotional state
Anticipatory	Occurring in advance	Anticipated fear
Chronic	Slow progression; long duration	Chronic gingival bleeding
Decreased	Smaller; diminished; lesser in size, amount, or degree	Decreased salivary flow
Deficit	Inadequate; not sufficient; incomplete	Knowledge deficit
Generalized	To extend throughout	Generalized gingival recession
Impaired	Made worse, weakened; damaged; reduced; deteriorated	Impaired dexterity
Increased	Enlarged; greater in size, amount, or degree	Increased plaque accumulation
Ineffective	Not producing the desired effect; not capable of performing satisfactorily	Ineffective plaque control
Localized depth	To confine to a definite place	Localized pocket
Potential	At risk; possible	Potential for infection

Table 3.4 • **ETIOLOGICAL FACTORS ASSOCIATED WITH DENTAL HYGIENE DIAGNOSES**

Problem		Etiological Factor
1. Xerostomia		Decreased salivary flow
2. Ineffective plaque control		Knowledge deficit
3. Increased plaque accumulation	related to	Impaired dexterity
4. Acute dentinal pain		Gingival recession
5. Potential for caries		Deep occlusal pits

condition. Sometimes a condition may be related to more than one etiological factor such as pregnancy gingivitis. This condition is dependent upon a pre-existing gingivitis and the hormonal changes associated with pregnancy. At times, the etiology will be unclear or unknown. It is acceptable to describe the problem using the words "related to unknown etiology" while continuing to search for the etiology. For example, alteration in comfort: pain related to unknown etiology. Table 3.4 lists some examples of etiological factors associated with dental hygiene diagnoses.

Dental versus Dental Hygiene Diagnoses

The dental hygiene diagnostic statement differs from the dental diagnosis, since it reflects the essence of dental hygiene rather than dental practice. The dental diagnosis identifies a specific illness, where the dental hygiene diagnosis identifies an actual or potential response to the illness. Dental diagnoses also suggest a dental need such as a restoration; dental hygiene diagnoses suggest a dental hygiene need such as diet modification, fluoride therapy, and alternative toothbrushing techniques. The purpose of the dental hygiene diagnosis is to direct dental hygiene treatment by focusing on the client's individual needs.

Guidelines for Writing a Dental Hygiene Diagnosis

Formulation of a dental hygiene diagnostic statement may be considered a new skill, however, the thought process has always been there. Like any new skill, this takes practice. The dental hygienist will find that, with practice, the process of writing dental hygiene diagnoses becomes easier.

The following guidelines have been adapted from the formulation of a nursing diagnosis and should be consulted when formulating dental hygiene diagnostic statements (Wilkinson, 1993).

1. Write the diagnosis in terms of response rather than need
2. Use "related to" rather than "due to" or "caused by"
3. Write the diagnosis in legally advisable terms
4. Write the diagnosis without value judgments
5. Avoid reversing the statement parts

6. Avoid including signs and symptoms of illness in the first part of the statement

7. The first part of the diagnosis should only include problems, or conditions

8. Be sure that the two parts of the diagnosis do not mean the same thing

9. The condition or etiological factors should be expressed in terms that can be changed

10. The dental diagnosis should not be included in the dental hygiene diagnostic statement

Each guideline will be discussed with examples. A table of incorrect and correct responses is included with most of the guidelines. As the clinician compiles this information, the formulation of dental hygiene diagnostic statements will take shape.

WRITE THE DIAGNOSIS IN TERMS OF RESPONSE RATHER THAN NEED

The first part of the diagnostic statement identifies the client's problem or concern. It can also be stated as a response to illness or state of health. Therapeutic or functional needs, such as "needs frequent fluoride therapy" or "needs flossing instruction," describe dental hygiene interventions rather than health responses and therefore should not be included in the first part of the diagnostic statement.

Example: Karen Alm is undergoing head and neck radiation therapy. She expresses the fact that her mouth and lips are dry. The dental hygienist concludes that she is uncomfortable because of dry mucous membranes caused by the radiation-induced decreased salivary flow. The dental hygienist communicates Karen's problems via the dental hygiene care plan in the diagnostic statement "alteration in comfort related to dry mucous membranes (xerostomia)."

Incorrect	Correct
Needs artificial saliva	Ineffective salivary flow related to radiation induced xerostomia
Needs fluoride therapy	Potential for root surface caries related to generalized recession

USE "RELATED TO" RATHER THAN "DUE TO" OR "CAUSED BY"

The two parts of the diagnostic statement should always be linked together by the words "related to." This identifies a relationship between the problem and the etiology and implies that if one part of the diagnosis changes, the other part may also change. "Related to" does not necessarily mean that there is direct cause and effect between the two parts. When such phrases as "due to" or "caused by" are used, the second part of the diagnostic statement could be interpreted as the specific cause of the problem. In reality, the dental hygienist may be unaware of other contributing factors that are influencing the condition.

Example: Bobby Vasko is six years old and afraid of the dental office. Upon examination, the dental hygienist assessed five restorations and one crowned tooth with root canal therapy. The dental hygienist identified multiple bad experiences as a contributing factor in his fear of dental procedures. Writing this diagnostic statement as "Fear of dental office caused by past dental experiences" implies that the multiple restorations are the cause of Bobby's fear. In validating this diagnosis, the dental hygienist discovers that Bobby's older brother constantly teases Bobby and describes the dental office as a place of pain. A more appropriate dental hygiene diagnostic statement is "Fear of the dental office related to past dental experiences and negative reinforcement."

WRITE THE DIAGNOSIS IN LEGALLY ADVISABLE TERMS

A diagnostic statement such as "potential periodontal pocketing related to incomplete scaling of calculus" is not legally advisable. This statement implies negligence or blame, which can create potential legal problems for the previous care provider. This statement could be better phrased as "potential periodontal pocketing related to subgingival deposit buildup." The dental hygiene plan of care or intervention would be similar in both instances, but the second statement does not imply fault and is still factual.

Incorrect	Correct
Potential for gingival abrasion related to inadequate use of air polisher	Potential for gingival abrasion related to hazards of air polishing

WRITE THE DIAGNOSIS WITHOUT VALUE JUDGMENTS

Dental hygiene diagnoses should be based on objective and subjective data collected and validated in cooperation with the client or significant other. The behavior of the client should not be judged by the dental hygienist's personal values and standards. Words such as inadequate, poor, and unhealthy are value judgments.

Incorrect	Correct
Increase in plaque accumulation related to inadequate home care.	Increase in plaque accumulation related to lack of knowledge regarding home care maintenance.
Disturbance in nutritional intake related to poor food choices.	Disturbance in nutritional intake related to knowledge deficit.

AVOID REVERSING THE STATEMENTS

Remember that the first part of the diagnostic statement reflects the problem and defines outcomes. The second part to the statement defines the etiology and suggests dental hygiene interventions. Reversing the statements may result in unclear communication about the client's problem and its etiology, making it difficult to write appropriate care plans. For example, the diagnostic statement "Generalized attrition related to grinding habit" is written so that the care plan goal is to reduce occlusal wear. The intervention associated with the second part of the statement or etiology is that the client will wear a night guard. If the statements were reversed, "Grinding habit related to generalized attrition," the goal may be to stop the grinding habit, but the intervention associated with generalized attrition is unclear.

Incorrect	Correct
Impaired mobility related to self care deficit	Self care deficit related to impaired mobility
High bacterial counts related to potential for infection	Potential for infection related to high bacterial counts

AVOID INCLUDING SIGNS AND SYMPTOMS OF ILLNESS IN THE FIRST PART OF THE STATEMENT

The first part of the diagnostic statement is derived from a grouping of signs and symptoms observed by the dental hygienist during the assessment of the client. An isolated sign or symptom is not a dental hygiene diagnosis, but it may provide clues to help identify the problem. Inaccurate diagnoses may occur if the dental hygienist focuses on an isolated sign or symptom rather than the entire clinical picture.

Example: Melissa Khan is 21 years old and presents for an oral examination. The dental hygienist observes that she doesn't smile and avoids showing her teeth. Writing the diagnosis as "Disturbance in self-esteem related to client's unwillingness to smile" suggests that self-esteem is the problem. In fact, the presence of not smiling may be a clue to other conditions such as fear, anxiety, extrinsic stains, or halitosis.

THE FIRST PART OF THE DIAGNOSIS SHOULD ONLY INCLUDE PROBLEMS

In some instances, clients express feelings regarding their illness or environment that are not necessarily unexpected or problematic. For instance, frustration may be an expected client response at a certain point in the process of treatment.

Example: Rhonda Jefferies is a 40-year-old social worker who presents with active periodontal disease in pockets 4 mm to 5 mm generalized throughout the mouth. She has received four treatments and is religiously performing her home care practices. At the time of evaluation most of her pockets remained the same. She was frustrated by all the time and money she invested and no reward (pocket depth reduction). Her frustration at this point is not necessarily inappropriate, therefore, it would be valid to write a dental hygiene diagnosis of "ineffective coping related to feelings of frustration." However, if later in treatment, Rhonda refuses to perform home care practices or skips appointments, her frustration does represent noncompliance, since it interferes with her treatment and maintenance.

BE SURE THAT THE TWO PARTS OF THE DIAGNOSIS DO NOT MEAN THE SAME THING

In some instances, diagnostic statements are written in which the two statements say the same thing. Examine this statement: "Inability to brush teeth related to oral home care problems." Both parts of the statement have the same meaning. In reality, the client is experiencing a problem in dexterity. The diagnostic statement should be written as "Ineffective oral home care practices related to limited dexterity."

Incorrect	Correct
Potential for root exposure related to areas of gingival recession	Potential for root exposure related to incorrect tooth brushing

THE PROBLEMS OR ETIOLOGICAL FACTORS SHOULD BE EXPRESSED IN TERMS THAT CAN BE CHANGED

Keep in mind that the diagnostic statement identifies actual or potential problems. These problems and the factors that contribute to their presence should be changeable by intervention within the realm of dental hygiene care.

Example: Jorge Rodriguez is examined following periodontal surgery and complains of tooth sensitivity. The diagnosis "alteration in comfort related to periodontal surgery" is not accurate, because dental hygiene interventions cannot change the position of the surgically replaced gingival tissue. However, the diagnosis can be restated as "alteration in comfort related to the effects of periodontal surgery." This statement allows the dental hygienist to intervene with desensitization procedures, fluoride therapy, and instruction for use of desensitizing home care products, which may relieve the effects of surgery—increased tooth sensitivity.

Incorrect	Correct
Alteration in oral mucous membranes related to oral cancer	Alteration in mucous membranes related to chewing tobacco
Potential for increased periodontal pocket depth related to gingivitis	Potential for increased periodontal pocket depth related to increased plaque accumulation

THE DENTAL DIAGNOSIS SHOULD NOT BE INCLUDED IN THE DENTAL HYGIENE DIAGNOSTIC STATEMENT

Two types of errors can be made when involving the dental diagnosis. The first is the use of the dental diagnosis in either of the two parts of the dental hygiene diagnostic statement. Since the dental diagnosis suggests dental interventions, its use is inappropriate in a dental hygiene diagnosis. The second type of error is a tendency to write the dental hygiene diagnosis as a paraphrased dental diagnosis. Although there is overlap in the dental hygiene and dental professions, the purpose of a dental hygiene diagnosis is to keep the planning of care focused on problems or conditions that are amenable to dental hygiene interventions.

Example: The statement "Potential for infection related to impacted third molar" contains a dental hygiene problem, "potential for infection," and a dental etiology, "impacted third molar." Therefore, the intervention associated with the etiology would be to extract the third molar, a dental intervention.

Incorrect	Correct
Potential for infection related to impacted third molar	Potential for infection related to plaque accumulation under operculum
Food impaction related to new three-unit bridge	Food impaction related to knowledge deficit of pontic debridement

During the formulation of the dental hygiene diagnosis, situations may arise that indicate more than one problem or etiological factor. It is important to combine these findings into one concise statement. Try to avoid writing wordy diagnostic statements or multiple statements with the same problem (or) etiological factor. See Table 3.5 for a listing of sample dental hygiene diagnostic statements.

Table 3.5 • SAMPLE DENTAL HYGIENE DIAGNOSTIC STATEMENTS

Oral hygiene
1. Generalized brown stain related to smoking
2. Potential for halitosis related to plaque accumulation on tongue

Intra oral
1. Black hairy tongue related to incorrect use of hydrogen peroxide rinses
2. Buccal mucosal ulcerations related to cheek biting

Extra oral
1. TMJ disturbance related to oral habit
2. Chronic lymphadenopathy related to partial third molar eruption

Dental Exam
1. Localized tooth sensitivity related to exposed root surfaces
2. Generalized dental abrasion related to incorrect toothbrushing

Periodontal Exam
1. Potential for periodontal infection related to high levels of periodontal pathogens
2. Altered bone level related to active periodontal condition

Medical History
1. Possible contact dermatitis related to allergic response to latex
2. Increased bleeding potential related to daily use of aspirin

Nutrition
1. Maxillary incisal decay related to improper bottle feeding pattern
2. Generalized erosion related to frequent regurgitation.

Personal Profile
1. Anxiety related to dental phobia
2. Body image disturbance related to discoloration of teeth

Finally, once all the pertinent factors in the diagnosis have been considered, the hygienist must determine the possible correlation of factors in the diagnosis. These relationships are often the key to effective treatment planning, since some problems must be addressed simultaneously to correct them, and other problems respond better if they are dealt with in sequence. The sequence itself is often critical, since problems addressed in the wrong sequence may lead to failure of treatment.

Summary

The dental hygiene diagnosis is part of the process of care. It is regarded as the thought process or bridge between assessment and care planning. During this phase data is classified, interpreted, and validated. Diagnostic statements are formulated to help the dental hygienist focus on the individual needs of the client. Following the dental hygiene diagnosis, a care plan can be devised that will address each individual need. Remember, the goal is to establish and maintain a healthy oral environment.

REFERENCES

Darby, M.L. (1990). *Theory development and basic research in dental hygiene: Review of the literature and recommendations* (1989–90 ADHA Council on Research). Norfolk, VA: School of Dental Hygiene, Old Dominion University.

Gordon, M. (1987). *Nursing diagnosis: Process and application* (2nd ed.). New York: McGraw-Hill.

Paul, R. (1988). *The critical student and person.* From the Eighth Annual and Sixth International Conference on Critical Thinking and Educational Reform. Rohnert Park, CA: The Center for Critical Thinking and Moral Critique, Sonoma State University.

Taptich, B., Iyer, P., & Bernocchi-Losey, D. (1989). *Nursing diagnosis and care planning.* Philadelphia: W.B. Saunders.

Taylor, C., Lillie, C., & Lemone, P. (1993). *Fundamentals of nursing* (2nd ed.). Philadelphia: J.B. Lippincot Publishers.

Wilkinson, J. (1993). *Nursing process in action.* Redwood City, CA: Benjamin/Cummings Publishing Company, Inc.

Exercise 3.1   Components of the Dental Hygiene Diagnostic Statements

Choose the most likely etiology for each of the following client problems from the numbered list.

	Problem		*Etiology*
_____	1. Potential for dentinal hypersensitivity		A. Plaque accumulation
_____	2. Altered nutritional status		B. Margination
_____	3. Gingival hyperplasia	related to	C. Knowledge deficit
_____	4. Potential for recurrent decay		D. High level endotoxin
_____	5. Increased periodontal pocket depth		E. Toothbrush abrasion

Exercise 3.2   Formulation of Dental Hygiene Diagnostic Statements

Write a dental hygiene diagnostic statement for each of the following assessment findings.

A. A teenager has a high plaque index score for interproximal surface areas. Client stated was never taught how to floss.

B. Client's teeth are sensitive to cold. Localized gingival recession.

C. Elderly client has arthritis in both hands. High levels of soft and hard deposits present.

Exercise 3.3   Identification of Assessment Findings

List the assessment findings one would expect to find given the following diagnostic statements.

1. **Diagnostic Statement:**
   Altered alveolar bone level related to active periodontal condition.

   Assessment Findings: _____

   _____

   _____

2. **Diagnostic Statement:**
   Chronic lymphadenopathy related to partial third molar eruption.

   Assessment Findings: _____

   _____

   _____

3. **Diagnostic Statement:**
   Maxillary incisal decay related to improper bottle feeding.

   Assessment Findings: _____

   _____

   _____

CHAPTER 4

Dental Hygiene Care Planning: Behavioral and Clinical Considerations

Learning Outcomes

At the completion of the chapter the reader should be able to:

1. Identify four stages of planning
2. Discuss how the use of the epidemiological approach assists care planning
3. Identify three levels of prevention and their application to dental hygiene practice
4. Describe three theories of health behavior and their implications for the development of the care plan

INTRODUCTION

The professionally educated dental hygienist has the ability to assess, critically analyze, and make sound judgments. In assessing the client's condition, the hygienist gathered information that led to a description of the client's current condition. In the identification process, conditions were differentiated as those that would benefit from dental hygiene therapy and those that would need dental treatment or treatment by other health professionals. The decisions were based on the dental hygiene body of knowledge and experience. The dental hygiene diagnosis focused on the current or potential disease states. Once the assessment and identification phases are complete planning can start. The planning component consists of four stages:

1. Setting priorities. Decision-making and negotiation skills are necessary to develop priorities with the client.

2. Developing outcomes. The ability to define goals and write behavioral objectives directs the desired outcome and the timeframes in which the goals will be reached.

3. Dental hygiene care plan. This stage culminates the planning process. It specifies the who, what, when, where, how, and the frequency of the planned activity.

4. Documentation. This stage is a byproduct of writing the individualized care plan and will occur simultaneously with the writing of the plan. It communicates the continuity of care and the planned evaluation.

To plan dental hygiene care, a foundation of current scientific knowledge and an understanding of behavioral theories is essential. After a short time in practice the hygienist can gauge fairly accurately how long the assessment of a client will take. Depending on the office procedures and the individual hygienist's skills, a thorough assessment of a new client may take from forty-five to ninety minutes. The planning phase is not as easy to quantify. Some clients with simple problems and clear preventive health values will require only a few minutes of discussion and education. Others will require a lengthy case presentation, education and counseling, and behavior modification or habit control. The more the hygienist knows about care planning, decision making, case presentation, and disease etiology and treatment, the more efficiently the planning phase will proceed.

The purpose of the planning phase is to identify the actions and interventions that will be most effective in rectifying the problems and producing the desired outcome. The plan will address two distinct areas that will be carried out in the implementation phase. The first is *clinical.* Those actions that the hygienist performs on the client in the office setting, such as quadrant root planing, require agreement from the client but leave the client in a passive state. The second area is *behavioral* and involves the client to a greater degree in the oral care plan. In both cases the client must be an active participant in the formulation of the plan and the decision-making process. The plan, no matter how well thought out with the best clinical and scientific judgment, will be doomed to failure if the client is not an active participant in devising the plan.

To help plan the types of interventions the hygienist and client will perform, the hygienist must not only have current scientific and clinical knowledge but also have an understanding of health behaviors and decision making.

The discussion of planning will be divided into two chapters. The first will discuss the types of prevention using the epidemiological approach and review three theories of health behavior. It will address the first stage of the planning process, setting priorities. The second chapter will introduce decision-making techniques in the complexity of care planning, development of outcomes as part of the care plan, and documentation, which are the three subsequent stages of the planning process.

CLINICAL CONSIDERATIONS OF PLANNING

The Epidemiological Approach

Hygienists educated in the United States and Canada for the past several decades have taken courses in community health and epidemiology. The most common working definition of *epidemiology* is "the study and effects of disease in populations over a period of time." This definition is based on the application of the scientific process and systematic observation of the innate nature of disease by searching for a cause. Generally we may think the principles of epidemiology as applied to populations would have little benefit in a private practice setting. However, epidemiology uses individual cases to develop hypotheses. Risk factors are identified, and symptoms are categorized and linked to possible or probable outcomes. That approach has given us the information we currently use as the basis for dental hygiene diagnosis and treatment. The hygienist who practices clinically with individual clients uses the broad base of scientific knowledge and then reverses the epidemiologic process, taking the information back to the source—the host/client. By integrating the two processes the hygienist can make both quantitative and qualitative judgments to plan current and future care. As care is planned, the dental hygienist must classify the stage of the client's disease, the risk factors that effect the course of the disease, and other host/client factors that may affect the course of the disease and/or impact on the types of interventions or protocols that can be applied to eliminate, reduce, or limit the course of the disease.

The *natural history of disease* (Figure 4.1) is a term used for over a century as an analogy for the clinical course of disease. Disease progresses from susceptibility, presymptomatic, and clinical to the final stage of disability. At the point of disability, the medical model delineates outcomes as "care," "cure," or "die." Obviously, in dental hygiene, "die" is fortunately a rare outcome. But conversely it is unfortunate that "cure" is also not as common as we would wish, leaving "care" as the most frequent outcome.

Another public health tenet that assists our decision-making/planning phase is the concept of levels of prevention. The levels of prevention are primary, secondary, and tertiary. Primary prevention occurs before the disease is present, secondary prevention is early diagnosis and screening, and the third level of prevention is rehabilitation of chronic disease and disabilities (Figure 4.1).

In the 1950s, Leavell and Clark (1953, 1965) formally designed a model to assist public health planners (Figure 4.2). This model divides the disease process into prepathogenesis and pathogenesis periods. The model is based upon some assumptions that focus on the vital aspects:

1. Health is a relative state. The authors of the model used the World Health Organization definition of health as "a state of total physical, mental, and social well-being, not merely the absence of disease or infirmity." The word "relative" means that everyone possesses some level of health and that a variety of factors, such as inherent or acquired characteristics and one's environment, affect the level of health.

2. Disease is a process. The disease process in humans depends on the nature and characteristics of the disease agents, and the individual's characteristics and response to stimuli. Health is a dynamic state, not static or stationary. Well-being fluctuates on a health continuum from optimum wellness to low-level wellness. Individuals function as a whole, with each dimension of health having an influence on others. Any physical illness, which most certainly includes the myriad of oral diseases, has an effect on the person's emotional well-being and social relationships.

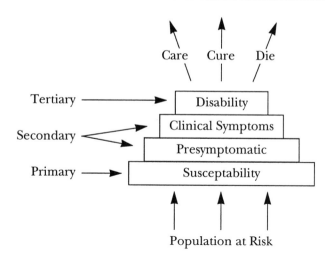

Figure 4.1 *Natural history of disease, with levels of prevention (Courtesy Leavell and Clark,* Preventive Medicine for the Doctor in His Community, *3E. New York, McGraw-Hill, 1965)*

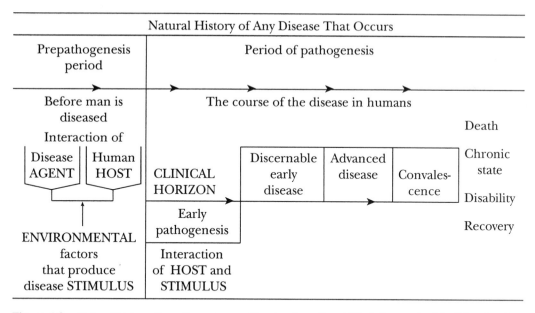

Figure 4.2 *Natural history of any disease process (Courtesy Leavell and Clark,* Preventive Medicine for the Doctor in His Community, *3E. New York, McGraw-Hill, 1965)*

3. Disease can have multiple causation. The level of wellness is a result of constantly interacting forces. Occurrence of disease is dependent on the triad of factors of host, agent, and environment. The *host* is the individual client; the *agent* may be chemical as in an aspirin burn, mechanical as in toothbrush abrasion, or biological as in juvenile periodontitis or moniliasis. *Environment* is an aggregate of all external conditions and influences affecting the life and development of the host, such as poor oral hygiene in relation to periodontal disease, lack of fluoride in the diet in relation to caries, or poor access to care posed by economic, political, and geographic barriers. This confluence has been called the "web of causation," which requires a susceptible host, a causative factor or factors, and an environment that is conducive to the interaction of host and agent. *Biologic gradient* is another term used to describe the susceptible host. It addresses the factor that individuals, even those with similar genetic backgrounds, have varying degrees of response to disease. It can be frustrating to the health educator to have one sibling who attempts to comply with all your oral health recommendations and continues to have less than the perfect checkup, while the other sibling seems to comply poorly and yet exhibits no disease.

According to the model, *prepathogenesis* is the predisease stage and may vary in time, beginning with the initial contact of host, agent, and environment and ending just short of the point when the disease can be objectively or subjectively detected. Other terms that describe this period could be incubation period or prodromal stage.

The *pathogenesis or disease period* begins at the point the disease can be clinically detected. This stage lasts until the host recovers, is disabled, or dies. The levels of prevention can be sequenced to coincide with the predictable events within each stage. Applying the correct level of prevention requires anticipation of future events based upon scientific knowledge of the natural history of the disease process. Increased epidemiological data and technological advances have brought us to the point that we can predict with some degree of certainty the course of the disease. For instance, based on DNA testing, bacteriologic assays and various clinical indices, we are able to assign periodontal disease to one of a number of possible stages and plan interventions appropriate to that stage. Time and host response continue to be factors that are not measurable and remain "best guess" based on epidemiological data and clinical experience. But there is no longer any excuse to plan client care based merely on protocol or subjective evaluation.

Levels of Prevention

There are five distinct types of preventive health practices within the three levels of prevention. Jong (1993) delineates each type of preventive dental service in four categories of oral disease: dental caries, periodontal disease, oral cancer, and oral-facial defects. He stresses the need to use this format to select priorities for the expenditure of money and other resources for community programs. However, the same needs exist for individual preventive care planning.

PRIMARY PREVENTION

Primary prevention strategies are aimed at preventing the initial contact of Host-Agent-Environment (H-A-E) (Figure 4.3). If there is no interaction, then the disease will not occur. The two types of primary prevention are *health promotion* and *specific protection*. Educational efforts are aimed at clients in the prepathogenic stage of disease.

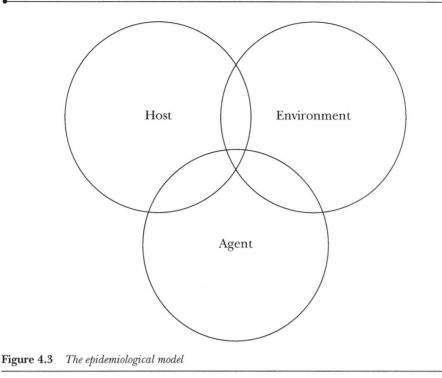

Figure 4.3   *The epidemiological model*

Health Promotion   Health promotion is aimed at a general well-being, making people aware of healthful practices and good hygiene. The goal of health promotion is to increase awareness and general knowledge. It differs from health education, which has a definite goal of a specified measurable change in knowledge, behavior, or attitude. Examples of health promotion range from classroom or group oral health presentations to television advertisements about oral care products. On the individual level, the hygienist may talk in general terms about an oral health topic to plant an idea in the client's head. Bille (1981) termed this *therapeutic seeding.* Learning occurs when the individual is ready or feels the need to learn. Seeding gives the client time to think about the idea and question on a subsequent visit. *Readiness to learn* is another term used in health behavior education. Since the client must accept responsibility for any behavior change, he or she must accept the challenge of learning and the effort of initiating the change. Once that point is reached then health promotion ends and true health education begins.

Specific Protection   Specific protection utilizes measures that will alter at least one aspect of the H-A-E interaction. Protection against accidents by using mouthguards for sports, fluoride programs, genetic counseling, or space maintainers are all areas of primary prevention.

SECONDARY PREVENTION
The purpose of secondary prevention is to diagnose disease at an early stage, slow progress of the disease, and prevent complications. Most of our efforts in periodontal disease are in this stage.

Early Diagnosis and Treatment   Careful assessment techniques enable early detection of oral disease that promote the reversal or halting of the disease. Incipient caries treated with a regimen of fluoride and improved diet combined with proper oral hygiene may prevent the decalcification process. Detecting gingivitis and intervening to alter the client's self-care can return the client to gingival health. Periodic reassessment and evaluation appointments that maintain the client's condition are another example in this category.

TERTIARY PREVENTION

The emphasis in this stage is on rehabilitation and disability limitations. The interventions are late in the pathogenic stage.

Rehabilitation   Full or partial prosthetic appliances, implants, and speech therapy are components in this category.

Disability Limitations   The purpose at this phase is to prevent or delay the consequences of the clinically advanced disease. The H-A-E has interacted at this stage and the goal is to minimize the pathogenic effects of the disease. Restorations, curettage, root planing, and root canal therapy all fall within this category.

CONSIDERATION OF H-A-E FACTORS

Epidemiological data has also taught us that a variety of factors increase a person's susceptibility to disease. We can evaluate each aspect of the triad for possible interventions. Before making any attempt to categorize risk factors, three points must be mentioned. First, not all risk factors are subject to change. Age associated with root caries, for instance, is unalterable. Second, even when strong statistical evidence suggests a link, not all individuals will develop the condition. Individual differences in response to disease stimuli, described earlier as the biologic gradient, make definite predictions unlikely. Third, in the brief description that follows the reader will see that there can be some overlapping of risk factors that make the decision about whether the influence is agent, host, or environment somewhat controversial. Presence of plaque is an example. It could be classified as a host factor because the individual uses poor hygiene measures, the agent because the bacterial content is causing gingivitis, or the biologic environment. There may be implications for all three. Although examples will be given for each category to help clarify the concept of risk factors, the reader should not be overly concerned with categorization. The important point to remember in helping to plan care is the confluence of those three circles (Figure 4.3). Where they come together to influence the disease process will help determine the care plan, set goals, and focus education and behavior change. Table 4.1 summarizes the application of preventive measures, based on the levels of prevention discussed above.

Host Risk Factors   A myriad of factors can affect the host's susceptibility to oral disease. Some factors may be inherent, such as genetic background, diseases such as diabetes, malocclusions, or lack of systemic fluoride during tooth development. Others can be acquired, such as inappropriate nutrition, poor oral hygiene, over-

Table 4-1 • **LEVELS OF APPLICATION OF PREVENTIVE MEASURES IN THE NATURAL HISTORY OF DISEASE**

LEVELS OF PREVENTION

PRIMARY		SECONDARY		TERTIARY
Health Promotion	Specific Protection	Early Diagnosis and Prompt Treatment	Disability Limitation	Rehabilitation
Preventive maintenance	Oral hygiene practice	Self examination	Scaling and curretage	Maxillofacial surgery
Periodic oral examination	Fluoride application	Screening examination	Periodontal surgery	Fixed and removable prosthetics
Dental health education	Mouthguards	Biopsy	Selective extraction	Implants
Anti-smoking campaigns	Smoking cessation	Provision of scaling and root planing	Chemo-therapy radiation	Speech therapy
Advertising	Lip sunblock use	Restorations	Major orthodontics	
		Minor orthodontics	Corrective maxillofacial therapy	
			Splinting and root resection	

hanging margins of restorations. Level of health knowledge, values, and attitudes are also factors.

Agent Risk Factors   Agent risk factors most obviously include the many bacteriological agents in the patient's oral cavity. Recent advances in periodontal research have categorized bacteria into destructive and nondestructive rankings. Additional research in root surface caries has also separated caries-causing bacteria. But an agent could also be the toothbrush in abrasion or high carbohydrate diet in rampant caries.

Environmental Risk Factors   There are three categories of environmental risk factors: biologic, socioeconomic, and physical. Poor plaque control measures, use of certain drugs, and xerostomia could fall into the biologic category. Poor access to care due to economic constraints or lack of adequate facilities or personnel due to political or geographic barriers can increase the environmental risk factors.

Once again the point is to use this helpful tool to focus thinking on identification of the etiology and contributing causes of the current or potential condition.

USING THE EPIDEMIOLOGICAL APPROACH TO PLAN CARE

The dental hygiene care plan is based on the problems identified in the diagnosis phase that are amenable to dental hygiene therapy. Dental hygiene interventions may be the only course of treatment the client will receive at this visit or series of visits, or they may be part of a broader dental care plan of treatments. It is crucial to identify those areas that are most efficiently treated by the hygienist to eliminate costly duplication of services and permit the dentist to devote time and expertise to those restorative, rehabilitative, or advanced periodontal treatments requiring those clinical skills. The working relationship within the office is critical to effective care planning.

Using the natural history of disease model, the hygienist determines if the client is in the prepathogenic stage or is exhibiting symptoms of pathogenesis.

The current scientific approach to assessment of the client's periodontal health uses the *specific plaque hypothesis.* In the past, dental hygiene therapy was based on nonspecific plaque removal, meaning that the concern was the amount of plaque. It was originally thought that more plaque led to increased disease. It was later realized that quantity of plaque was not the central issue—thus arose investigation into specific microorganisms and their roles in the oral environment. Additionally, host response, or stated differently, one's immune response to the bacterial invasion, determines the course of the disease. Environmental factors such as smoking affect the host's susceptibility and suppress the immune response. Systemic factors, such as diabetes or positive HIV status, use of steroidal compounds or other pharmacological preparations as exemplified by phenytoin, are further examples of factors that affect the host's immune response. As we approach the twenty-first century, dental hygiene treatment modalities address tissue response to the interventions, rather than simply the evaluation of calculus, plaque removal, and root smoothness. As the clinician begins to analyze and synthesize the data from the client's assessment, he or she must keep all current concepts in mind.

Collecting the clinical data described in Chapter 2 will enable classification of disease. To review, the data collection includes history-taking, gingival and periodontal clinical assessment, intra and extra oral examination, and a radiographic survey as a minimum baseline. To be thorough, it should also include such diagnostic tools as gingival crevicular temperature and/or fluid samples. Bacterial plaque can be analyzed by DNA probes or cultures. Enzyme tests and DNA assays, currently being developed or new to the market as of this writing, provide additional information with relative ease and at a minimal cost. It is the professional's responsibility to be knowledgeable about current modalities of data collecting and identification.

Nearly all oral conditions will have a dental as well as a dental hygiene diagnosis. Some conditions will require treatment provided solely by the hygienist, but many oral conditions will be treated jointly by the dentist, hygienist, and/or other health professionals.

Defining Characteristics of Disease

To illustrate how this process works, consider the male client in his early twenties who comes to the office complaining of sore bleeding gums and is scheduled with the hygienist. The first thing noted is a malodor from the his mouth, although he is well groomed and neatly dressed. The client's chief complaint is pain, bleeding, and halitosis, with an inability to eat. The initial intra/extra oral exam indicates lymphadenopathy, and the client's skin feels warm to the touch. The gingival assessment reveals ulcerated papillae with a pseudomembranous covering. The slightest manipulations cause bleeding. Probing is too painful for him to tolerate. Visible supragingival calculus is seen on the maxillary molars and mandibular anteriors. The classification of this condition would most likely be necrotizing ulcerative gingivitis (NUG). We know this because the *defining characteristics* of the disease were listed. The defining characteristics of a disease are the clinical signs and symptoms, or the findings of various diagnostic tests. Some defining characteristics, such as sulcular bleeding, may be linked with more than one disease, such as gingivitis and periodontitis. Additional defining characteristics would help describe the disease: Bone loss would differentiate gingivitis from periodontitis. The next step in formulating a dental hygiene diagnosis and subsequent care plan would be to assess the *contributing or risk factors*. Risk factors can be defined as characteristics that are associated with an increased rate of disease or disability. It is a disease precursor and can include everyday health practices, family history, demographic variables and some physiologic changes. Traditionally, NUG has been associated with mental or physical stress, with predisposing factors of poor oral hygiene. Conceivably in the future new research may link specific immunological deficits caused by stress, but currently stress is considered to be a defining characteristic. The etiological factor to consider is HIV status.

The *dental* diagnosis would focus on the gingivitis and its treatment, which would include initial palliative treatment provided by the hygienist and possible antibiotic therapy. The *dental hygiene* diagnosis, however, will look more holistically at the client, striving to identify the associated risk factors. The client should be counseled by the hygienist and/or the dentist to seek HIV testing if he has any high risk behaviors. Since test results take some time, treatment would continue.

Some professionals may view recommending HIV testing as a second stage diagnostic tool used if the client does not respond to initial therapy.

The dental hygienist would describe the client as follows:

> Bleeding, pseudomembranous, ulcerated gingiva. Calculus visible near salivary ducts. Client reports stress of finals and studying for graduate school entrance exams. Client exhibits lymphadenopathy and appears febrile.

Due to the severity of the condition, the hygienist will want to consult the dentist for possible antibiotic therapy and confirmation of the disease diagnosis. Decision of the immediate course of action would then be decided.

Contributing Factors

The hygienist then must consider the known contributing factors of the disease that are related etiologically or contributory. Those factors could be considered from two aspects:

Pathophysiological: All those factors that are physiological in nature, such as amount of deposit, and those that are pathologic, such as bacterial levels and types

Psychosociobehavioral: All other types of factors, including anxiety and stress, pain tolerance, lifestyle, and oral hygiene practices

The risk factors are then identified. In the abbreviated assessment, calculus was noted as were the swollen glands and fever. All these were pathophysiological. The psychosociobehavioral factors for this client include anxiety and stress, poor oral hygiene practices, possibly fear or lack of knowledge. Inadequate nutrition, lifestyle orientation, and reduced financial access to dental care are all factors that may predispose the current condition.

The dental hygiene diagnostic statements will address the current condition and appropriate risk factors. The care plan will define the specific interventions and their frequency that the hygienist and/or the client will perform as well as the expected outcome of each. The dental hygiene diagnoses for this client would be:

1. Inability to eat related to bleeding, pseudomembranous, ulcerated gingiva

2. Risk for impaired healing related to poor oral hygiene practices

3. Knowledge deficit regarding oral hygiene practices

4. Alteration in nutritional needs related to current lifestyle

5. Feelings of anxiety and stress related to current lifestyle

For each diagnostic statement the hygienist would plan the interventions and state the expected outcomes as the projected care plan. In the acute stage the expected outcomes would be short-term. As the condition improves some reassessment may be in order. The client needs to be involved in any goal setting, either short or long term. An individual in acute distress only wants relief from those symptoms as quickly as possible. To discuss altering lifestyle for this client, for instance, would be futile at this time. The empathetic plan addresses immediate needs and concerns. The client recognizes that sensitivity and will be more likely to be receptive to further interventions and education at subsequent appointments.

BEHAVIORAL CONSIDERATIONS OF CARE PLANNING

To discuss planning thoroughly it is necessary to review some of the theories of health behavior and health education. The three theories that will be discussed are the *health belief model*, the *multiattribute theory*, and the *human needs model*. The clinician must have a working knowledge of health behaviors and must apply a combination of theories to guide in the development and evaluation of the planned intervention. Understanding the social-psychological basis for health behavior helps to direct the education and facilitate the strength of the chance for lasting change.

Health Belief Model

OVERVIEW
The health belief model (HBM) was developed in the 1950s by a group of social psychologists at the U.S. Public Health Service. Although it has undergone some revisions since its inception, it remains one of the few social-psychological theories directed solely at health behavior. The HBM grew out of the confluence of two theories that were being used quite extensively at the time: the Stimulus-Response (S-R) Theory (Hull, 1943) and the Cognitive Theory (Lewin, 1935).

Briefly, S-R theorists believe learning results from events called reinforcements that produce a drive that activates behavior. Cognitive theorists place a high value on the mental processes of thinking and reasoning. Both believe that the reinforcements or consequences of behavior operate by influencing the expectations or value of the outcome, thereby directly influencing the behavior.

The HBM theorizes that individuals will take preventive health action if they believe that

1. they are susceptible to the condition;
2. the condition has serious consequences;
3. they can take actions/interventions that will be beneficial in reducing either the severity or susceptibility to the condition; and
4. the benefits outweigh the perceived barriers such as time or cost or other negatives.

Other variables have also been applied. The one most accepted is that educational attainment has a direct influence on preventive health behavior, thus increasing the likelihood of utilizing preventive health services and or/taking other preventive health actions. Therefore, the higher a person's education the more likely he or she will follow recommendations.

APPLICATIONS TO DENTAL HYGIENE

Perceived susceptibility   This is a subjective perception of one's own susceptibility. It can work positively when the client recognizes that initial signs and symptoms indicate early disease and statistically it would be likely for him or her to get the disease. Conversely, it can also work negatively if the client is somewhat fatalistic—"Everyone in my family has that problem, and there isn't anything I can do about it."

Serious consequences   Since dental disease rarely has life-threatening implications and most periodontal disease is a slow, chronic condition with no startling symptoms, some clients may not perceive the severity of oral diseases without some education. Others who place a high value on maintaining a healthy oral environment will want to discuss the consequences of treatment.

Benefits of Intervention   The client must believe that a certain behavior, either his or hers in self-care regimens or the practitioner's via clinical treatment, will lead to the expected outcome. Another aspect that has more recently been incorporated into the HBM is called *self-efficacy*. The individual must believe not only that the intervention is efficacious, but that he or she can execute or perform the behavior. The problems in modifying long-term behavior and incorporating behavior change into one's lifestyle must be surmounted by the individual. In short, the client must feel confident and competent to implement the change.

Perceived Barriers   What may be a barrier to one individual is not to another. Time and money are two perceived barriers that readily come to mind in that context. One client may feel that the cost of treatment is prohibitive while another is more concerned with the time it will take.

Due to its wide acceptance, the HBM has been used as the basis for many studies. One review article (Janz and Becker, 1984) examined over one hundred studies using the HBM in the ten-year period preceding publication of the article. All support the model as being a good predictor of health behavior with the most powerful predictors being "perceived benefits" and "perceived susceptibility." On the negative side is the comment that beliefs in themselves are not a sufficient cue to action and that attempts to change beliefs are difficult at best. Some behaviors, such as toothbrushing, have such a habitual component that influencing change in style or frequency is very difficult.

APPLICATIONS TO THE CARE PLAN

The clinician can assess each of the components of the HBM with a few questions or careful listening during the assessment phase. Vulnerability can be ascertained and evaluated by asking some questions that test the client's "dental IQ" and then linking the response to the actual data in the assessment. Perception of severity can be evaluated by the client's attitude to pain or tooth loss, or how much he or she values keeping his or her own teeth.

Perceived benefits can be measured at the same time by listening carefully to the responses to judge the value placed on maintenance of oral health. *Locus of Control* is another concept that describes how individuals handle situations. A client who feel powerless to do anything about a situation, that his or her condition is due to bad luck, genetics, or previous circumstances is said to be an "external"—control of the situation is external to this person. These individuals are less likely to manage change without close monitoring and extensive counseling. The "I-can-do-it" kind of client is internally controlled, easily motivated, and more likely to be susceptible to change attempts. Recognizing these differences in individuals will help to determine the degree of authority or control the clinician should assume at the onset of a planned program of change. An internally controlled client would more readily accept self-monitored change that he or she can manage with less direct supervision. Teaching the client how to monitor change or do a self-exam, or providing a small dental mouth mirror will encourage the new behavior. On the other hand, the externally controlled person may feel overwhelmed by the responsibility and feel inadequate to do what he or she sees as the professional's job. More time is needed to make this person self-sufficient. Frequent maintenance, assessment, and/or evaluation appointments are called for with the client who believes he or she has less control over his or her health. Your own orientation towards your interpersonal relationships with clients needs to assessed to evaluate the degree to which you exhibit control.

The issue of self-efficacy must also be addressed. Rosenstock, Strecher and Becker (1988) indicates that "in the realm of chronic disease control, much more emphasis is likely to be needed on skill training to enhance self-efficacy. Specifically, self-efficacy can be enhanced by breaking the complexities of the target behavior into components that are relatively easy to manage." He further cautions that it is necessary to identify the specific aspects that require skill development. "Specific behaviors must then be arranged in a series so that they can be consecutively mastered, with initial tasks being easier than subsequent tasks." Self-efficacy can also be enhanced by setting short-term goals toward the ultimate long-term goals. Successes can be reinforced by praise; lapses are viewed as an opportunity to analyze and subsequently control the factors that caused the lapse. The methods involved in self-efficacy will be further discussed in Chapter 6, Implementation.

Multiattribute Utility Theory

OVERVIEW

The effectiveness of interventions to encourage a client to change behavior is determined to a great extent on identifying the major concerns and barriers preventing the change. If the health educator emphasizes topics that are of no interest or have little relevancy to client, change will be unlikely. The multiattribute utility theory (MAU) provides a method of systematically identifying those issues that are important to the individual.

MAU is based upon *value expectancy theories* that provide a framework for systematically evaluating the issues involved when an individual must decide a specific course of action. The value of an outcome can be stated objectively, in terms of cost-saving measures, or subjectively in terms of feelings, as exemplified by the client's making healthful diet choices as the "right" decision. Values that individuals hold about health-related issues greatly affect their willingness to seek health care and follow therapeutic regimens. Value expectancy theory asserts that the health-related behavior is the result of a *value* that the person places on the outcome of an action and the individual's *expectation* that the action will indeed lead to a desired outcome. The health belief model and locus of control concept are actual examples of a value expectancy applied to health situations. A value is more than a belief or an attitude. It is a standard or criterion used by the individual for the purpose of making evaluations. Values are abstract ideals held by the person. Family security, a sense of accomplishment, independence, self-discipline, capability, and social recognition are all examples of values.

MAU predicts behavior directly from an individual's evaluation of the consequences or outcomes associated with either performing or not performing a behavior. The MAU theory provides a methodology for breaking complex decisions into individual attributes—the consequence, outcome, or cause. For instance, we frequently assign attributes to everyday occurrences. At the first sign of a cold many people will assign the origin to a recent event ("I got wet and chilled in that rainstorm the other day."). That attribute is based on the belief held by the individual. As with many beliefs, scientific evidence that points to the contrary is simply ignored. The belief is: If I get wet and chilled I will likely get a cold. The *value* the person puts on the interventions will tell us something about that person's expectancies. If the person does nothing and gets "lucky" by not having a cold develop, he or she may hold an external locus of control. On the other hand, if the same person acts by taking additional vitamin C, getting extra rest, and so forth, that person may be internally controlled. Additionally, the HBM could be applied to the scenario as the belief that a cold would be serious enough for the person to take active preventive measures. Notice at this point that we are not judging the value of the belief, which may or may not have a basis in fact, but rather the value expectancy. In breaking the complex issue into areas of concern, the decisionmaker (client) can evaluate the strengths of each attribute. Weights are put on each attribute that are used by the health educator to predict the likelihood of the behavior's taking place.

APPLICATION OF MAU TO THE CARE PLAN

The classic use of the theory was used to determine the feasibility of taking a flu shot. When making such a decision we may view our choices of getting the disease or not. If we win the gamble we may say we were lucky, but if we lose we may end up quite ill, lose time at work, or even run the risk of giving the disease to others. If we decide to take the flu shot, we may end up with some discomfort, possibly even a mild case of the flu. Plus we have to go through the hassle of appointment making and scheduling. Using MAU theory the individual would list the pros and cons for each attribute. Each of these statements is then assigned a weight. The individual gives each attribute a score, with the most important receiving ten, and the lease important one. An attribute of "lost time at work" may receive a seven, while "giving the flu to others" be given a ten if a medically compromised family member lives in the home. It is important that the individual make differentiations between those concerns that are important and those that are not. It forces the person to seriously weigh the consequences of acting or not. Research has indicated that the model is predictive of behavior, with 82 to 87 percent actually taking the shot (Carter, 1992).

We may apply this theory to clients in an informal way when giving oral hygiene instruction and attempting to initiate new self-care routines. Many failures in changing client behavior result from assumptions on the part of the clinician about the individual's attitudes, value, or concerns.

Weinstein, Getz and Milgrom (1985) identify a number of problems that contribute to why plaque control programs don't work. They believe that most programs begin too early, before the clinician gets to know the client, and programs fail unless the client assumes ownership of the problem. Another important aspect of failure is that the professional makes assumptions about the client's nonperformance that are often mistaken. Until we address the issues of concern to the client, we may be wasting time. We need to hear what the client thinks are the pros and cons. For a decision about a complicated or costly course of treatment, it may be worth applying the MAU theory to its fullest—having the client explore his or her concerns with you and ranking or weighting them. If time doesn't allow, or the client is resistant to the technique, ask questions that focus on identifying some concerns. "How important is (issue) to you?" can be asked. Issues can be time, money, fear of discomfort, or opinions of others. Once pros and cons are identified, then effective interventions can be planned.

In private practice the dental hygienist sees many clients who are well past any primary preventive measures. A client who is in Stage III or IV Periodontitis will be required to make some very important decisions. The professional should help the client identify the issues that are of concern. Proceeding with a course of treatment may include fear of surgery and pain, cost, or appearance. Refusing surgery may mean more frequent recalls to slow the progress of the disease, extractions, loss of function and appearance. This is a big decision for the client, not a simple "either/or" choice. There are many ramifications, including health, work, and leisure-related activities, social concerns, and appearance. Some attributes, such as appearance, might fall under both pros and cons in the weighting. Helping the client identify those attributes about the decision that are personally important will enable you both the find the correct choice of action. Figure 4.4 illustrates some of the issues that may be discussed. There may be more pros than cons or vice versa in a person's list. This division itself may be revealing to the client, immediately identifying that there are more reasons to do something than not. There are more attributes listed in Figure 4.4 under the "having surgery" side than the other. Until the client differentiates the pros from the cons, however, we don't know what is important and what is not.

Remember, it is important to force the differentiation and weighting. They cannot all receive a score of ten.

Many people do not have good decision-making skills. In addition, when faced with decisions deemed serious or threatening, such as surgery or extractions, the individual may react emotionally. It is incumbent upon the professional dental hygienist to develop skills that encourage clients to make well-thought-out decisions.

Human Needs Conceptual Model

OVERVIEW

Probably the best known human needs theorist is Maslow. Maslow's hierarchy of needs seen in model form is a triangle with physiological needs at the base. Pro-

NO SURGERY

Health 1 2 3	Activities 4 5	Attitudes 6 7 8 9 10
1. Current/future discomfort 2. Complications 3. Losing function of teeth	4. Cost of full or partial replacements 5. Extractions - lost time at work	6. Appearance 7. Halitosis 8. Other's opinions 9. Wearing dentures 10. Frequent recall to forestall additional problems

SURGERY

Health 11 12 13	Activities 14 15 16	Attitudes 17 18 19 20
11. Discomfort 12. Complications 13. Keeping oral function	14. Lost time at work 15. Cost 16. Scheduling surgery	17. Appearance 18. opinion of others 19. Keeping up with maintenance 20. Self care requirements

Figure 4.4   *MAU taxonomy of client periodontal decisions*

ceeding up the triangle are the needs of safety and security, love and belonging, self-esteem, and finally self-actualization at the apex. Maslow theorized that a hierarchy means that lower order needs must be satisfied before the higher order can be met.

Recently in dental hygiene literature Darby and Walsh (1993) conceptualized a dental hygiene process model based upon the human needs model as adapted by Yura and Walsh (1988). They indicate that the Maslow categories were too broad in scope and the structure too limiting to apply well to dental hygiene care. Ambiguities existed in applying certain dental hygiene actions such as prophylaxis or etiological relationships to Maslow's structure. Yura and Walsh's human need theory was adapted for nursing and includes human needs categories articulated by Maslow but arranged differently, supplemented with those that facilitate clinical assessment. Yura and Walsh identify thirty-five human needs, grouped into areas of survival, closeness, and freedom needs. Dental hygiene theorists had by this time espoused the concept of defining the domains of dental hygiene practice to include client, environment, health/oral health, and dental hygiene actions. These concepts were accepted by the American Dental Hygienists Association in 1993 and were defined in Chapter 1. According to the model, the dental hygiene process—comprised of assessment, analysis, planning, implementation, and evaluation—of care is at the core.

Darby and Walsh (1993) validate eleven of the thirty-five human needs as applicable to dental hygiene. The following section identifies those needs and gives a capsulized version of their application to dental hygiene.

APPLICATION OF NEEDS TO DENTAL HYGIENE

1. *The human need for safety is defined as the need to experience freedom from harm, or danger involving the integrity of the body's structure and environment around the person* (Darby and Walsh, 1993). Any health deficit that may interfere with or compromise dental hygiene care may threaten the client's safety. These can include elevated blood pressure, the need for prophylactic antibiotics, or the client's concern about infection control. The hygienist must assure the client that every effort is being made to ensure comfort and safety.

2. *The human need for wholesome body image is defined as the need to have a positive mental representation of one's own boundary and how it looks to others* (Darby and Walsh, 1993). Much of this has to do with self-concept. Concern about the appearance of one's teeth, facial profile, or any facial disfigurement relate to body image. Compliments and assurances can help the client focus on positive attributes. Assisting the client to find other support systems when needed for rehabilitation are a responsibility of the hygienist.

3. *The human need for freedom from pain/stress is defined as the need to be exempt from physical and emotional discomforts* (Darby and Walsh, 1993). The hygienist needs to use pain control measures appropriate for the client, and when necessary refer clients to programs of control for detrimental oral habits, substance abuse, or chemical dependency, including tobacco use.

4. *The human need for skin and mucous membrane integrity of the head and neck is defined as the need to have an intact and functioning covering of the person's head and neck area—including the oral/mucous membranes and gingiva—which defend against harmful microbes, provide sensory information, and resist injurious substances and trauma* (Darby and Walsh, 1993). The hygienist's attention is directed to intra/extra oral lesions and gingival and periodontal health. Thorough periodontal care provided by the dental hygienist and/or referral to other periodontal specialists meets this need.

5. *The human need for a biologically sound dentition is defined as the need to have intact teeth and restorations that defend against harmful microbes and provide for adequate function and aesthetics* (Darby & Walsh, 1993). The hygienist must include a complete examination, record findings, and note deviations from normal. Clients need to be counseled regarding the use of fluorides and sealants and other preventive measures that assure a healthy dentition.

6. *The human need for nutrition is defined as the need to ingest and assimilate sufficient amounts of carbohydrates, proteins, fats, vitamins, minerals, trace elements, and fiber required for growth, repair, and maintenance of structurally and functionally component* *body parts* (Darby and Walsh, 1993). Clients need to receive specific instruction for diets that are conducive to oral health. Those with rampant caries or other oral conditions linked to inadequate nutrition need diet analysis and counseling.

   7. *The human need for conceptualization and problem-solving is defined as the need to grasp ideas and abstractions, to reason, to make sound judgments about one's life and circumstances* (Darby and Walsh, 1993). The hygienist needs to explain rationales and methods for prevention, correct misconceptions, and create relationships of abstractions to the client's reality.

   8. *The human need for appreciation and respect is defined as the need to be acknowledged for achievement, worth, service, or merit and to be regarded favorably with admiration and approval by others* (Darby and Walsh, 1993). The hygienist must establish positive interpersonal relationships with the client to meet this need.

   9. *The human need for self-determination and responsibility is defined as the need to exercise firmness of purpose about one's self and accountability for one's behavior and actions* (Darby and Walsh, 1993). Clients need to be fully involved in goal setting and self-care.

   10. *The human need for a value system is defined as the need to have an internalized designation of the importance of people, institutions, things, activities, and experiences in one's life* (Darby and Walsh, 1993). The hygienist needs to attempt to identify what the client values and build on that. Those with a low priority for health will challenge the hygienist's ability to educate for health-promoting behaviors.

   11. *The human need for territoriality is defined as the need to possess a prescribed area of space or knowledge that a person denotes as one's own, maintains control over, defends as necessary, and is acknowledged by others as owning* (Darby and Walsh, 1993). The hygienist needs to be aware of nonverbal as well as verbal cues related to personal space and privacy. Clients need to be assured of confidentiality.

APPLICATIONS TO CARE PLAN

Using the human needs model for planning care, the hygienist would assess each of the needs to determine if there are any deficits. If there are, then interventions are planned. For example, if the client comments that he or she is dissatisfied with discolored teeth, that person has a deficit in body image, defined above in need 2. The hygienist must then determine if the discoloration is intrinsic or extrinsic, and whether dental hygiene interventions alone, such as scaling and polishing, will rectify this problem or whether dental interventions such as bleaching or laminates will be required. The dental hygiene diagnosis would be: Human need deficit in wholesome body image related to self-image of discolored dentition.

USING THE THEORIES TO PROMOTE BENEFICIAL HEALTH BEHAVIORS

Developing Therapeutic Relationships

Determining the client's locus of control may be the first step in understanding his or her role in the care plan. As previously mentioned, external attributes include luck, clarity of directions or previous education, quality of previous care, family, and environment. The extent to which the individual feels in control of these circumstances determines his or her internal locus. If an individual with a strong internal locus has failed in previous preventive attempts, his or her self-esteem has been lowered. Internals may also have difficulty dealing with chronic disease states, since they feel they have lost control. Knowledge of a client's attributions or perceptions of important and mitigating factors allows the hygienist to tailor language detailing the important aspects of education and treatment to the client's needs. It is very important that explanations be clear. Using analogies that help understanding and eliciting frequent feedback to see that the message is understood are essential.

Changing incorrect or negative attributions will most certainly test the clinician's ability. The goal must be to replace a negative attribution with an alternative. If the client failed in previous attempts, the focus of dental hygiene education should be identifying those external events that were specific at that time. Focusing on those unstable events means that the change was not achievable at that time. By identification of those circumstances, the hygienist and the client can focus on planning what will ameliorate or eliminate those barriers or skill deficits, thus promoting a more likely successful outcome. If the client has incorrect information, education directed at the correct or current thinking needs careful direction away from judgmental references.

THE ROLE OF INFORMATION IN HEALTH-RELATED DECISIONS

Accurate knowledge is critical to making a decision, but is not sufficient in itself to promote a change in behavior. It is particularly evident when communicating the what, when, where, and how of performing actions. Much consumer research has been conducted that indicates the consumer seeks to process as little information as possible to reach decisions quickly. We can all think of exceptions to this rule, surely, and therefore we need to identify the few who want to do careful research before making a decision. However, the majority of people use "satisfying" rather than "optimal" as a criterion. The consumer may not continue to search for the *best* alternative if he or she is satisfied with the alternative that suits them as being hassle-free with the least disruption to their lifestyle.

Consumers apply *heuristics*, which are guidelines. A heuristic could be, when in doubt, choose the cheapest, or the nearest, or even the most expensive. The simple solution may not be the best. The clinician must be ready to guide the client to make the best possible choice at the current time. Information should be *readily available*. Product information, efficacy of treatments, and the clinician's success rate or experience are in this category. The information must be *useful*, yielding new insights about the product, service, or behavior. The information must be *processable* within the client's limits of time, energy, and comprehension. When speaking with the client, an image of a knowledgeable, up-to-date professional must be portrayed. Use of statistics regarding products such as saying "Brand X reduces 80 percent of the harmful bacteria" rather than "Brand X works well" is more effective. Frequency of performing treatments and the level of experience is also assuring. Indicating statements such as "in the ten years I've practiced" or "in the dozens of cases I've treated that were similar to yours" help the client recognize expertise. One can be an authority without being authoritarian, and confident without being a braggart. The client wants to feel that the practitioner they have chosen is the best and by communicating expertise trust is enhanced. One caution is to tell the truth. Be accurate in your statements and don't overestimate either your own ability or the success rate of treatments.

Summary

To start the planning process, the dental hygienist must have a broad background in the biomedical and behavioral sciences. Current knowledge of oral disease, its classifications, signs, symptoms, and treatment protocols is a critical foundation for planning. Technical knowledge alone, however, will not help the client if the clinician's interpersonal skills, including a deep understanding of human behavior, are not strong. Preventive health behavior is a complex issue that continues to challenge the most experienced practitioners. For many, it is this part of dental hygiene practice that creates the greatest challenge and therefore produces the greatest rewards.

REFERENCES

Bille, D. (1981). *Practical approaches to patient teaching.* Boston, Mass: Little and Brown.

Carter, W. (1992). Psychology and decision making model: Modelling health behavior with multiattribute utility theory. *Journal of Dental Education, 56,* pp. 800–807.

Darby, M. and Walsh, M. (1993). Application of the human needs conceptual model of dental hygiene to the role of the clinician: Part II. *Journal of Dental Hygiene, 67,* pp. 335–346.

Hull, C. (1943). *Principles of behavior.* Norwalk, Conn: Lange.

Janz, N. and Becker, M. (1984). The health belief model: A decade later. *Health Education Quarterly, 11,* pp. 1–47.

Jong, A. (1993). *Community dental health,* St. Louis, MO: Mosby.

Leavell, H. and Clark, E. (1953, 1965). *Preventive medicine for the doctor in his community.* New York, NY: McGraw-Hill.

Lewin, K. (1935). *A dynamic theory of personality.* New York, NY: McGraw-Hill.

Rosenstock, I., Strecher, V., and Becker, M. (1988). Social learning theory and the health belief model. *Health Education Quarterly, 15,* pp. 175–183.

Weinstein, P., Getz, T., and Milgrom, P. (1985). *Oral self care: Strategies for preventive dentistry.* Reston, VA: Reston Publishing Company.

Yura, H. and Walsh, M. (1988). *The nursing process, 5 ed.* Norwalk, Conn: Appleton and Lange.

Exercise 4.1 Levels of Prevention

Identify the levels of prevention (primary, secondary, and tertiary) and their sub-categories (i.e., specific protection) for each of the following:

_____ 1. Sealants

_____ 2. Oral self-examination

_____ 3. Fluoride therapy following radiation treatment for head and neck cancer

_____ 4. Dietary counseling for a client with rampant decay

_____ 5. Myofunctional therapy

_____ 6. A dental hygiene table at a health fair sponsored by the local component of the American Dental Hygienists' Association

_____ 7. An oral health screen at a local nursery school as part of an overall health awareness day

_____ 8. Detection of a small raised white lesion on the client's palate.

Exercise 4.2 Differentiating Defining Characteristics and Risk Factors

For each of the descriptions listed, place a check mark in the appropriate category.

Description	Defining Characteristic	Risk Factor
Sulcular bleeding		
Poor oral hygiene		
Excessive exposure to sun for fair-skinned individual		
Use of juice bottle at baby's bedtime		
High sucrose intake		
Decay of maxillary central incisors of a 3-year-old		
Elevated diastolic blood pressure reading		
Mottled enamel		

Exercise 4.3   Applying Multiattribute Theory

List as many attributes as you can think of for the following situation:

A 26-year-old single female elementary school teacher must make a decision regarding orthodontic treatment. She has been told that her current occlusion is contributing to the headaches and TMJ dysfunction she is experiencing. She also feels that her crowded lower anteriors and lingually placed lateral incisor are detrimental to her smile. Her case will require an estimated twelve months of orthodontic intervention requiring bands, and the wearing of a palatal appliance for at least one year following removal of the bands. Her dental insurance does not cover orthodontic treatment for adults, and the estimated cost of the treatment is $2500.

The hygienist in this office does a portion of the initial intake appointment, including history taking, impressions, radiographs, and charting before the orthodontist sees the client for the initial examination. When the client returns for the second case presentation visit, the client meets with the hygienist first and views commercial videotape presenting information about adult orthodontics, some situations that the client can expect to encounter, some of the limited risks, and finally the benefits of treatment. The hygienist then answers questions and talks to the client prior to the dentist's case presentation.

Questions:

1. Help the client identify the attributes. Putting yourself in the client's place as much as you possibly can, list eight or more pros and cons to starting treatment. Limit your list to no more than fifteen.

2. Weighting. To each of the pros or cons give a weight, using a maximum of ten for those important, a one for those least important, and a range in between. Anything with a weight of 8 or more is a serious consideration.

3. Making choices. Those attributes that are weighted heavily on the "con" side should be examined to see if any planning or intervention can be instituted to render them less important. They should be also compared against those that are similarly weighted in the "pro" category to assist in the decision.

CHAPTER 5

Developing the Dental Hygiene Care Plan

Learning Outcomes

At the completion of the chapter the reader should be able to:

1. Identify care plan alternatives that correlate with client expectations
2. Determine the appropriate goals, interventions, and expected outcomes associated with a dental hygiene diagnosis
3. Identify the components of an expected outcome statement
4. Design an individualized dental hygiene care plan based on the dental hygiene diagnosis
5. Prepare a detailed appointment plan that indicates number of visits, time for each visit, and associated interventions

INTRODUCTION

Dental hygiene care plans are designed to promote quality care by facilitating individualized care, continuity of care, communication, and evaluation. The information contained in the care plan should clearly communicate the client's specific needs and effective strategies to manage them. The plan acts as the blueprint or roadmap for describing the who, what, when, where, and how of the treatment so that implementation and evaluation are not haphazardly performed.

As discussed in Chapter 4 the first step in care planning is establishing priorities: what needs must be addressed first, second, third, and so on. These priorities are based on the dental hygiene diagnosis. The next step in care planning is identifying the alternatives. There are many ways to reach the established goal, and by identifying the alternatives the hygienist will be able to design the most appropriate care for the client. Finally, after determining which alternatives are most likely to achieve the desired results, the expected outcome is written in terms that define what the client and caregiver are required to do.

Writing the care plan involves stating the desired goals as they relate to the dental hygiene diagnosis, developing the dental hygiene interventions that will achieve the desired goals, and formulating the expected outcomes. Following the care plan, the appointment plan is developed by sequencing and organizing the dental hygiene interventions into specific appointments.

IDENTIFYING ALTERNATIVES

Developing alternatives requires the clinician to categorize dental hygiene therapy into the areas of clinical and behavioral interventions and to view disease as prepathogenic or pathogenic in order to begin to define the roadmap for care. When planning a trip an individual may opt for a circuitous, longer route for any number of reasons. It may be more scenic, or convenient to stop and see a friend along the way. Others may choose the fastest or the cheapest route. Depending on all the contributing factors an individual may choose one route one time and an alternate route some other time. In short, no decision can be made until all the options are weighed for that specific time—how much time or money are available, the reason for going, and less measurable, but probably the most important, the person's individual style or desires. Consider the analogy to dental hygiene care planning. Just as all but the most experienced traveler will generally use a travel expert (agent) or a mapping service to guide their decisions and trip, the hygienist must see him- or herself in the role of oral health expert honestly offering alternatives and exploring possibilities. It would be ludicrous for a travel agent to "hard sell" a luxurious cruise vacation to someone who would rather hike and camp in the mountains. In a similar situation, the hygienist must also listen to the client's desires and past experiences. The ideal treatment envisioned by the hygienist will not be successful if it is in conflict with the client's perception of ideal. Do not confuse the client's desires or lifestyle with his or her ability to pay. To continue the analogy, people of moderate means may save diligently for an occasional luxury vacation, while another more affluent person may opt for a simple vacation or even stay at home. The clinician must take care not to make stereotypical judgments. The point of this analogy is that the hygienist must constantly remember individual differences, respect others' values and keep his or her own subjective opinions in check.

Let us now consider the hygienist who after an hour of careful assessment of a new client has determined the dental hygiene diagnosis and is ready to formulate the care plan. If the practice policy uses a separate appointment for case presentations, then alternative treatments should be presented at that time. If the dental hygiene care plan is presented to the client at the diagnostic appointment, then discussion of alternatives with the client should start as soon as they are formulated. All the previous categories discussed—behavioral, clinical, pathogenic, prepathogenic, classifications of periodontal disease and so forth—help to focus on the possible routes and alternatives to optimum oral health. If a client is in an acute state, choices are most likely limited. Most clients, however, will present in asymptomatic, preacute, or chronic states. Those individuals are the ones who present the challenge to planning and are the greatest bulk of the clinician's client population.

Influencing a Client's Behavior Choices

Logan (1991) delineates two routes through which an individual can be persuaded. One route is said to be *central* and the other *peripheral*: "The central route emphasizes the information a person has about the issue under consideration. Persuasion under this route is based on careful and thoughtful consideration of the arguments presented and occurs to the extent that the data are integrated into a reasoned position" (p. 570).

If the central route is followed, the person has thought deeply about the topic. Research indicates that the attitude is more long-lasting, predictive of behavior, and it is harder to dissuade the person (Cacioppo and Petty, 1981).

Conversely, the peripheral route is based less on a thoughtful interpretation of the issues and more on external cues related to the argument, such as grammar, dress or demeanor of the speaker, promise of reward, or the surroundings. In this route, behavior is unpredictable, the message is easily forgotten, the attitude is vulnerable to counterpersuasion and will continue only as long as the cues are salient.

What this research says is that the source of the message can be more important than the message itself to many people. In addition, unless a client is considering a lengthy and/or expensive course of treatment, he or she may consider much of what you say irrelevant and therefore follow a peripheral route. If that is the case, then not only expertise but also the manner of presentation and interpersonal skills are critical. The quality of the message is rated by the individual on the strength of the argument. Characteristics of strong versus weak and plausible versus implausible are the judging factors. Strong arguments will require factual scientific information indicating efficacy of recommendations. This also satisfies one of the health belief model tenets. The client must believe that he or she is not only susceptible, but that action on his or her part will have a benefit. The second judging factor of plausible/implausible is one of issue involvement or personal relevance. The issue must have personal importance or meaning or satisfy an intrinsic value.

Many current dental hygiene texts refer to fear arousal techniques as being poor motivators. Insufficient research has been done in dental care settings to support this popular belief. On the contrary, research in other medical settings indicates moderate fear arousal messages can be effective strong arguments for the possibility of the recipient's suffering negative consequences (Petty and Cacioppo, 1981). Many hygienists may not be using this tool if they are not honestly portraying the likelihood of serious consequences of oral neglect. Additionally, moderate anxiety arousal can facilitate message reception. Texts have also cautioned against trying to persuade anxious clients. An individual who is moderately anxious about a current or potential condition is more likely to be ready to accept involvement in a care plan.

The Chinese have a saying: "If you give a starving man a fish you will keep him from starving for one day, but if you teach him to fish you will keep him from starving for life." That proverb is similar to the professional value of dental hygiene. Instructors in schools of dental hygiene start modeling preventive thinking to their students by explaining, the dental hygienist doesn't "clean" teeth, the client "cleans" his or her own teeth. The hygienist provides education and periodontal maintenance therapy.

The professional dental hygienist needs to examine his or her own values. If the primary professional value is to educate the client for self-care and independence, then understanding the process of critical thinking and decision making is essential. The terms are not synonymous. Critical thinking will enable the clinician to weigh the alternatives. It presupposes an in-depth knowledge of the disease process, classification of disease, and the usual protocols to meet those needs. It is a reasoning process that requires the clinician to look for alternatives that are not rigid and allow for individual differences. It enables the clinician to establish the dental hygiene diagnosis and to begin to formulate the dental hygiene care plan. The decision-making process enables the client and the hygienist to implement the plan.

To return to the analogy of trip planning, we need to decide which way we will go on the trip, how long we will take to get there, what preparations we will have to make, how much money we will be able to spend, and any contingency plans for possible mishaps. Good planning need not be lengthy or time consuming. The more one uses the process has a positive effect on reducing the time it takes to plan. The only critical thing about planning is when the decision-making process occurs. It must be at the outset. Too often we forge ahead with little thought to the outcome of our endeavors and end up spending more time making corrections or failing in the attempt altogether. There is a "pop-culture psychology" that promotes "positive thinking." While much can be said for that attitude, it is not an excuse for ignoring the reality of a situation.

One tool for making decisions is the "what if" game. Some might start a trip with bald tires on the car and, if luck holds, may make the destination without mishap, but *what if* the tires fail? We could use an either/or approach: buy new tires/don't buy new tires. If we buy new tires, the pro is that we don't have to worry about the tires failing, but the con is that we'll have less money for the trip. If we don't buy the tires, we'll have that money, which is good, but maybe we'll end up spending more on the road if we need to buy new tires. We could also think of some contingency plans. Each person faced with this scenario will weigh the alternatives based on innate attitudes (i.e., are they risk-takers?) and on past experience.

More important, however, would be the central issue: Why am I making the trip? If it's a vacation, then maybe it will have to be postponed; but if it's essential, for instance to visit a sick relative, that changes how the alternatives will be evaluated. When we make decisions we need to develop options based upon the goal. The options should be creatively developed, not an either/or possibility. If our goal was to take the trip to see a sick relative, one alternative solution might be to take a bus instead of one's own automobile. When looking at decision making, don't fall into the trap of setting a solution and then working backwards. The goal of issue identification is to answer the question "What am I really trying to accomplish?" Solutions that are win/win rather than yes/no, and are positive and preventive rather than reactive to the situation are the most effective.

To apply this concept to dental hygiene therapy consider the client whom you have assessed with three areas of pocket depths greater than 5 mm and some faulty bridgework. The client has fair oral hygiene, brushes regularly, but flosses only occasionally. The client is a businessperson with dental insurance that she notes "isn't too good." You additionally assess that the client has "moderate" concern for her optimum oral health on your personal scale of poor to excellent. The client's knowledge or dental IQ is quite high. How would you help this client make decisions that are meaningful? What issues or concerns will you need to focus on that will assist the client to a purposeful and thoughtful decision? Remember, your best or optimum treatment may not be the same as the client's.

With this client we need to explore the pros and cons, the "what if" choices. You will need to listen carefully to what the client views as "cons." Perhaps the client sees the need quite clearly for improved oral health, but is most concerned about costs because she currently has two college-aged children and tuition payments are a priority. Exploring alternatives with this client must focus clearly on the most cost-effective choices. Reviewing what the insurance will cover may be an early step. Carefully point out that home care preventive measures are low cost and effective. Seek alternatives with the client in ways to implement change in behavior that can be integrated into her lifestyle without creating a new chore. The hygienist needs to review what in-office dental hygiene therapy can be performed that will eliminate or control the etiology of her periodontal problems, and what dental interventions can contain the problems associated with the faulty bridge. Conversely, the client may be unconcerned or even resistant to any preventive efforts. The hygienist's goal may be trying to establish more frequent recall appointments, instituting a regimen of irrigation or antimicrobial rinses, and seeking ways to motivate the client to a more active role in disease control.

Seven Decision-Making Steps

There are seven steps to consider in making decisions.

1. What is the issue? Why is the decision necessary? What are the consequences of doing nothing?
2. State your purpose. Broadly determine what you are trying to achieve
3. Set your criteria. Specify how much you will do to reach your goal
4. Establish priorities. What are the most important or critical?
5. Search for solutions. How can you reach the criteria?
6. Test for alternatives. How does each solution meet the criteria?
7. Troubleshoot. What can go wrong?

Let's consider a common problem in dental hygiene practice. To the following case scenario we will apply the seven steps of decision making.

CASE SCENARIO

The client is a middle-aged businessman. He states he has tried flossing and absolutely won't do it. He continues to give you a litany of complaints about flossing, how it got stuck in between his teeth, how much time it took, and so on. He is adamant about not flossing, but not hostile.

This scenario identifies an assessment of the client's knowledge and skill concerning home care, specifically interproximal plaque removal. The dental hygiene diagnosis would be: Potential for interproximal bleeding related to a knowledge deficit of flossing alternatives. According to the diagnosis the care plan goal is "improved interproximal plaque removal."

1. What is the issue?

RDH: Let me ask you a few questions. When you tried flossing did the floss keep breaking between your teeth?

CLIENT: Yes, all the time. It would shred and get stuck and then I'd have to try to get it out with a tooth pick. It was a hassle.

RDH: Did it happen between all your teeth or just some of them?

CLIENT: Yeah, well, mostly the back ones.

2. State your purpose.

RDH: Mr. Milton, you know you are having some pocket formation and slight bone loss on those back teeth. I see in the chart the previous hygienist noted talking to you about this. I'd like to take a minute or two to explore some possibilities that may not have been discussed last time to help you remove the plaque in those areas.

CLIENT: Yeah, sure, but don't expect me to start flossing.

RDH: Sometimes when a person starts doing something different, it seems difficult. I understand that it feels frustrating to have so much trouble with something that seems like it should be so simple. Maybe last time all the problems and difficulties weren't explained and so you felt annoyed that you found it so hard to do. You know, there are many different kinds of floss; some are stronger than others and there are other ways to remove plaque from between your teeth.

CLIENT: Really. Like what?

3. Set your criteria.

RDH: Well, for one waxed floss or a different brand is stronger. Also sometimes it helps to pull the floss through in tight areas, rather than coming back up through the contact. We can evaluate how tight the contacts are between your teeth and check the x-rays to see if any fillings are catching the floss. And last, there are toothpicks or other devices that are some help. They may not be as effective as floss but they would be better than doing nothing. The question you will have to decide is how much time and energy you want to expend to get the results you want. We can tailor the solution to your needs. What we are really trying to achieve here is the reduction of the toxic effects of bacterial plaque. Those areas that can't be reached by a toothbrush continue to cause an inflammatory response of your tissue to those bacterial irritants. Anything you can routinely do to reduce the plaque helps to reduce those toxins.

CLIENT: Well, you know, I guess I never really thought about it in those terms. It just seems that flossing was such a hassle. But I really don't want to start losing any teeth or spending all my time at the periodontist. Okay, what are some of these other ways, I'm willing to listen.

4. Establish Priorities.

At this point the hygienist needs to determine with the client what his goal is—how much time and effort will he be willing to put into learning and changing his behavior. The hygienist should first try flossing his teeth with a sturdy floss to evaluate the tightness of the contacts and consult the radiographs to check for overhanging margins. If brushing is part of the problem, that needs to be addressed also.

5. Search for Solutions.

To build rapport, the hygienist can comment on the difficulty of some areas. She then asks the client to try several spots to determine dexterity. The conversation continues briefly, determining if dexterity is part of the problem. If so, a floss holder and strong floss might be the simple solution. A powered toothbrush might do a better job in a short period of time. This client seems concerned with time, so focusing on time-saving solutions in the short term are good points to make.

6. Test for alternatives.

If all of the flossing strategies are rejected and the client still says "No way," what then? Remember the goal is improved plaque removal, not perfect plaque removal. We may need to suggest toothpicks, rinsing with approved mouthwashes, or home oral irrigation as alternatives. The client needs to understand that these alternatives may not be as effective as flossing. Whatever the final plan, evaluation needs to be built at future appointments. We can be judicial in choosing our options and thus limit alternatives and be creative. We need to analyze the desirability of each action with the likelihood that it will be performed.

7. Troubleshoot.

Helping the client to identify the most troublesome areas, what to do if the floss gets struck, and which pharmacy near the office carries what you recommend are all enabling factors that contribute to the success rate of the planned program.

The entire process listed above takes no more time than any other educational intervention. The client was made to feel a part of the plan from the start. Empathy was established and the past experience was not judged as failure. The discussion focused on some of the client's values. The conversation revealed that the client had some knowledge of why flossing is necessary. The hygienist, however, successfully moved away from the importance of the task orientation to the goal of plaque removal. Once that aspect is presented the client may agree to going the "best" route of establishing flossing with some appropriate modifications rather than the easiest route of alternatives.

As we set the priorities, establish the criteria, and identify the alternatives we are beginning to define the care plan. For this case scenario, the care plan would involve teaching the client to use a floss holder or another interproximal oral physiotherapy aid such as a toothpick or oral irrigator.

WRITING THE CARE PLAN

The care plan is a written proposal based on the dental hygiene diagnosis. It contains three components: the overall goal, specific interventions, and the expected outcomes. The following will address each of these components and how they relate to the dental hygiene diagnosis. As a general guideline, the goal statement refers to the first part of the dental hygiene diagnosis, the problem. The interventions refer to the second part of the dental hygiene diagnosis, the etiology (Figure 5.1).

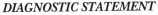

DIAGNOSTIC STATEMENT

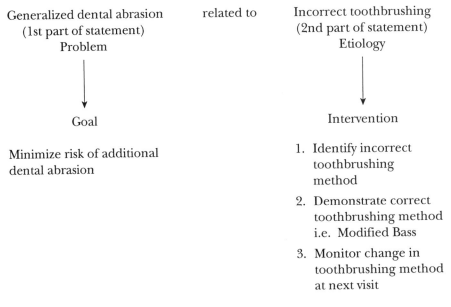

Generalized dental abrasion (1st part of statement) Problem	related to	Incorrect toothbrushing (2nd part of statement) Etiology
Goal		Intervention
Minimize risk of additional dental abrasion		1. Identify incorrect toothbrushing method
		2. Demonstrate correct toothbrushing method i.e. Modified Bass
		3. Monitor change in toothbrushing method at next visit

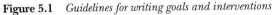

Figure 5.1   *Guidelines for writing goals and interventions*

Stating the Goal

Goal statements are used to identify the overall reason for care. They are broad statements about the desired effects of the dental hygiene interventions and are directly associated with the dental hygiene diagnostic statement. At least one overall goal statement should be written for each diagnosis. For example:

> *The Diagnostic Statement:*
>
> Potential for increased caries activity related to reduced ability to remineralize
>
> *The Care Plan Goal Statement:*
>
> Increase the tooth surface resistance to demineralization

The dental hygiene diagnostic statement identified the actual or potential conditions or behavior that in the clinician's professional judgment were considered to be a problem for the client. This then implies that an alternative behavior or treatment will be required to correct or ameliorate the problem. The goal statement described the overall desired result (see Table 5.1).

Dental Hygiene Interventions

Dental hygiene interventions are designed to assist the client in reaching the desired goal. They should be written in enough detail so that they can be interpreted by all caregivers. Dental hygiene interventions provide specific directions and instructions to the client and the clinician to eliminate or alter the etiological factors identified in the second part of the dental hygiene diagnosis. To achieve the final desired outcome, interventions, either clinical regimens or strategies of behavior change that address the problem, must be designed. For instance, the dental hygiene diagnosis is "Potential for increased caries activity related to reduced ability to remineralize tooth surfaces" by evidence of decalcification. The overall goal is to "Increase the tooth surface resistance to demineralization." Dental hygiene interventions need to be developed that answer the questions How do you assist in the remineralization of tooth structure? How do you decrease the

---

Table 5.1 • **SAMPLE GOAL STATEMENT**

Dental Hygiene Diagnosis:
Potential for decalcification related to green stain

Goal Statement

Increase tooth
surface resistance
to demineralization
and improve oral
hygiene

potential for demineralization? Some dental hygiene interventions that provide some answers are:

1. Dietary counseling
2. Plaque control education
3. Professional fluoride treatment
4. Home fluoride treatments with the use of a custom tray

Each of these interventions can be further broken down into specific tasks. For instance, intervention 4 (home fluoride treatments with the use of a custom tray) can be divided into four separate tasks:

1. Take an alginate impression for the development of a custom tray
2. Make a plaster model from the impression
3. Fabricate the custom tray
4. Educate the client in correct application of home fluoride therapy

The extent to which the steps of the dental hygiene interventions are described is determined by office protocol or the individual skill level of the clinician (see Table 5.2). For a student, it might be helpful to include as many steps as possible until protocol procedures become incorporated into his or her knowledge base.

Long-Term Goals and Short-Term Outcomes

Short-term outcomes give direction to the long-term goal. It may take weeks or months to achieve the desired result and therefore require a number of steps or short-term outcomes. It is both educationally sound and intrinsically motivating to

---

Table 5.2 • **SAMPLE DENTAL HYGIENE INTERVENTIONS**

Dental Hygiene Diagnosis:
Potential for decalcification related to green stain

Goal Statement	Interventions
Increase tooth surface resistance to demineralization and improve oral hygiene	1. Take plaque index and give plaque removal instructions, i.e., brushing, flossing 2. Fluoride OTC daily rinse 3. Polish green stain 4. Scale remaining areas of deposit 5. Apply in-office fluoride treatment NAF 6. Re-evaluate for decalcification three months

apply several short-term outcomes with degrees of difficulty that increase over time. The analogy can be made to the failed New Year's resolution that states, "I will lose twenty pounds" or "I will stop smoking." In general, statements that do not contain timeframes or have steps delineated along the way are doomed to failure, except for the most highly motivated and self-directed of persons. To be successful, a statement should specify the behavior or performance criteria and a target date. Second, each should have short-term achievable, self-motivating outcomes. It would be more realistic for the weight loss statement to say "in my goal of a twenty pound weight loss, I will lose eight pounds by January 31." Another strategy would be specify the behavior. To stop smoking, someone might start by cutting down, thus saying, "I will not smoke in the car for the next month." The same guidelines are applied to writing outcome statements with clients. Short-term outcomes may be a list of the clinical interventions you, as a clinician, will perform and those that the client agrees he/she will perform. You must both agree that the outcomes are achievable and appropriate for whoever is to perform them. Essentially, the expected outcomes along with the interventions become the treatment plan.

Stating the Expected Outcomes

Expected outcome statements are based on the premise that the statement should be concise, measurable, and understandable. A clearly written outcome statement enhances communication between client and practitioner, and between various practitioners. It also assures continuity of quality care.

Expected outcome statements should be

1. client-centered;
2. clear and concise;
3. observable and measurable;
4. time-limited;
5. realistic; and
6. determined by client and practitioner together.

CLIENT-CENTERED

An outcome statement is written to focus on the behavior the client is expected to perform. It must address what the client will do, when and/or where the activity will be performed, and the extent or frequency. An example is a diagnostic statement that identifies "gingival bleeding related to incomplete plaque removal." An outcome statement would be: "Reduce bleeding score by 50 percent in one week using the Bass method of toothbrushing and flossing daily."

CLEAR AND CONCISE

Standard terminology or abbreviations must be used. The statement should not be overly long but must be clear. The statement should not be ambiguous or open to various interpretations. "Effective plaque removal" for instance, can mean different things to different clients. Defining a percentage of reduction or a specific score is more precise. The "how" of the plaque removal should describe manual versus electric brush, proxibrush, or floss as examples.

OBSERVABLE AND MEASURABLE

The "what" is answered in this part. Words that describe feelings should be avoided. "Appreciates fresh breath," for instance, cannot be measured as an outcome for plaque removal on the tongue. Specifying how frequently a behavior should be performed or the extent to which the outcome can be measured in actual scores or percentages are essential elements of the outcome statement.

TIME-LIMITED

The timeframe of the outcome should be limited and in general be short. Most dental hygiene outcome statements will be stated in terms of days or a week or two. Some regimens may require one to three months. However, it should be remembered that although the ultimate goal may be a lifelong change, the outcome statement and interim visits should be scheduled for frequent feedback and monitoring.

REALISTIC

An outcome should be achievable without causing extreme changes at the outset, unless there is an acute problem. The client's readiness to change are affected by many factors. It is far better to set an expected outcome that is easy to attain and have the client achieve success then to have the client feel he or she has failed. Expectations can always be increased at re-evaluation appointments.

DETERMINED BY THE CLIENT AND DENTAL HYGIENIST

At the initial assessment the dental hygienist started involving the client by learning the client's views, attitudes, and values. Helping the client find the "right fit" in time, effort, and expenditures will improve success for both client and practitioner.

Guidelines for Writing the Expected Outcome

Each statement should contain a subject, an action verb, performance criteria and a target time (see Table 5.3).

Subject—The subject is a noun. It could be the client, a part of the client's body, or a property or characteristic of the client.

Examples: Mrs. Miller

Plaque

Stain

Inflammation

Action Verb—The verb describes what the client is supposed to do. The client is in a learning situation. Even if he or she knows how to do something reasonably

---

Table 5.3 • **GUIDELINES FOR WRITING EXPECTED OUTCOMES**

1 Performance	+	2 Conditions	+	3 Criteria	=	Expected Outcomes
What is the learner able to do?		Under what conditions will he or she do it?		How will he or she know when he or she has accomplished it? How well must it be done?		

Example 1 (Goal: Establish a habit)
Subject: The client
Performance: will brush his teeth
Conditions: using the Bass technique
Criteria: following each meal for three consecutive days.

Example 2 (Goal: Improve home care)
Subject: The plaque score
Performance: will be reduced
Criteria: by 75 percent
Conditions: at the following visit.

---

well, such as floss, this behavior has not been incorporated into the daily routine. Educational theorists have categorized learning into three domains: cognitive, psychomotor, and affective. *Cognitive learning* is an intellectual process that starts with fact gathering and culminates in appraisal and decision making. The second domain, *psychomotor learning*, primarily directs learning that involves some manipulative skill and physical ability. It also includes the perceptual abilities of visual and sensory discrimination. This can be important to remember as the client needs to use sensory cues to self-evaluate effectiveness of plaque control techniques. *Affective learning*, the third type, is most complicated to measure and the most difficult type of behavior to alter. It involves values and beliefs, feelings, attitudes, and compliance.

The choice of action verbs is important because it identifies what needs to be done and helps with future evaluations. Table 5.4 lists some words that have limited interpretations in each of the three categories. Terms such as "to know," "to appreciate," "to value," and "to understand" have multiple meanings and are very difficult to measure.

Performance Criteria—Performance criteria answer the questions of what, when, how, and where. They set a standard and describe the *extent* to which a client is expected to perform the behavior. It is the portion of the statement that enables evaluation.

It can address:

   Amount—will floss daily for one week

   Quality—will reduce plaque by 50 percent in one week

   Accuracy—will identify cariogenic foods in diet with 100 percent accuracy.

Table 5.4 • **ACTION VERBS USED WITH OUTCOME STATEMENT**

Cognitive	Psychomotor	Attitude/Affective
define	demonstrate	appraise
repeat	practice	evaluate
list	operate	choose
describe	measure	select
explain	assess	compare
plan	use	schedule
formulate	inspect	incorporate

Table 5.5 • **SAMPLE EXPECTED OUTCOME STATEMENTS**

Dental Hygiene Diagnosis:
Potential for decalcification related to green stain

Goal Statement	Interventions	Expected Outcome Statements
Increase tooth surface resistance to demineralization and improve oral hygiene	1. Take plaque index and give plaque removal instructions i.e., brushing and flossing 2. Fluoride OTC daily rinse 3. Polish green stain 4. Scale remaining areas of deposit 5. Apply in-office fluoride treatment NAF 6. Re-evaluate for decalcification	1. Decrease plaque score by 50 percent within one week 2. Demonstrate adequate toothbrushing and flossing technique on self 3. Record daily use of fluoride on index card 4. Visually assess complete removal of green stain 5. Tactilely assess remineralization of decalcified areas in one month

Target Time—Each outcome statement should have a target time in which we can realistically expect a change to occur. It helps to direct the future appointments, but more importantly is motivating to the client in achieving a certain level of change by a specific point in time. It also provides a timeframe or deadline for evaluation. Table 5.5 contains sample expected outcome statements.

APPOINTMENT PLANNING

Once the care plan has been established, the interventions need to be outlined in sequence. The sequence is then organized by appointments. If only one dental hygiene diagnosis is identified, and the interventions listed in the care plan can be accomplished in one appointment, then the appointment plan is comprised of the listed interventions. Note that the interventions listed in the care plan should be carefully sequenced. On the other hand, if there are multiple dental hygiene diagnoses and many interventions, the sequencing and organization of these interventions into the appointment plan becomes more complex.

The sequencing of dental hygiene interventions usually reflects the dental hygienist's philosophic approach to providing care. Woodall (1993) states that differences in philosophy are apparent among health care providers when deciding how to sequence preventive and therapeutic procedures. Some clinicians believe that ensuring the client's control of his or her oral health comes before most treat-

---

Table 5.6 • **SAMPLE APPOINTMENT PLAN**

Dental Hygiene Diagnosis:
Potential for decalcification related to green stain

Goal Statement	Interventions	Expected Outcome Statements
Increase tooth surface resistance to demineralization and improve oral hygiene	1. Take plaque index and give plaque removal instructions i.e., brushing and flossing 2. Fluoride OTC daily rinse 3. Polish green stain 4. Scale remaining areas of deposit 5. Apply in-office fluoride treatment NAF 6. Re-evaluate for decalcification	1. Decrease plaque score by 50 percent within one week 2. Demonstrate adequate toothbrushing and flossing technique on self 3. Record daily use of fluoride on index card 4. Visually assess complete removal of green stain 5. Tactilely assess remineralization of decalcified areas in one month

APPOINTMENT PLAN

Since there is only one dental hygiene diagnosis, the interventions are sequenced in the order in which they would be implemented at appointment #1. Therefore the appointment plan for appointment #1 would follow the intervention list in the care plan.

Appointment #2 (fifteen minutes/one week)
1. Take plaque index and compare to baseline score
2. Evaluate client's dexterity and skill level for plaque control procedures
3. Review plaque control regimen with client and check for any problems

Appointment #3 (fifteen minutes/one month)
1. Evaluate areas of decalcification
2. Take plaque index and compare to previous score
3. Review plaque control regimen with client and check for any problems

ment. Others believe that prevention should follow basic treatment procedures. However, most dental hygienists integrate preventive procedures into each appointment. Sequencing dental hygiene interventions is influenced by such factors as the status of the condition (acute or chronic), the severity of the condition, the extent of the condition, and the need for any special treatment precautions.

When developing the appointment plan and the sequence of specific dental hygiene interventions, it is helpful to review protocol. For instance, if the client is to be effective in plaque control, then access needs to be established by the removal of supra- and subgingival calculus deposits. Therefore, the appointment plan would require that scaling procedures be accomplished before the initiation of such home care procedures as flossing. Another example is a client who has an acute condition and is in need of subgingival debridement but is a dentophobic. In this case, before treatment procedures begin you must address the client's fear.

Estimating the time needed to perform each procedure and the time interval for evaluation will direct the number of required appointments. The amount of time needed will vary according to the clinician, client, and type of equipment available. Time management skills are developed throughout the dental hygiene educational process and are considered to be an important part of appointment planning. Table 5.6 contains a sample appointment plan.

SAMPLE DENTAL HYGIENE CARE PLAN

The following is a complete dental hygiene care plan, which includes the diagnosis, goal statement, interventions, expected outcomes, and appointment plan.

After the assessment of a 40-year-old woman, the dental hygienist formulated the following diagnoses.

DIAGNOSTIC STATEMENTS

1. Inflammed palatal mucosa related to improper denture care
2. Generalized gingival inflammation of anterior region related to lack of motivation of plaque removal

CARE PLAN

Diagnosis #1

Inflammed palatal mucosa related to improper denture care

Goal #1

Eliminate inflammation of palatal mucosa by instituting proper denture care

Interventions

1. Educate regarding negative consequences of not removing denture
2. Provide instruction for the daily care of dentures, i.e., soaking and cleansing

Expected Outcomes

1. Remove denture daily for six to eight hours
2. Soak denture in cleansing solution following removal
3. Return in two weeks for re-evaluation of palatal inflammation

Diagnosis #2

Generalized gingival inflammation of anterior region related to motivation of plaque removal

Goal #2

Prevent gingival inflammation through incorporation of effective daily plaque control

Interventions

1. Explain the effect of bacterial toxins on the gingival tissues via phase contrast microscope
2. Disclose plaque and take a Navy plaque index
3. Identify bleeding points on a bleeding index
4. Show progression of disease and premature aging as a result of further tooth loss
5. Evaluate client's home care regimen
6. Make corrections regarding modified Bass toothbrushing method and flossing

Expected Outcomes

1. Demonstrate a 50 percent reduction in both plaque and bleeding index scores in two weeks
2. Record daily home care on index card
3. Client will inspect disease status by use of disclosing solution and presence of bleeding (pink toothbrush)

APPOINTMENT PLAN

Appointment One (one hour)

1. Educate regarding consequence of not removing denture
2. Take plaque sample and with the use of a phase contrast microscope describe the effects of bacterial toxin on gingival tissue (Note: the technique for using the phase contrast microscope can be identified in the intervention section of the care plan or in the appointment plan if necessary)
3. Explain progression of disease—tooth loss
4. Describe the correct sequence of denture care
5. Take plaque and bleeding index
6. Evaluate present home care regimen

7. Educate on proper toothbrush and flossing techniques

8. Antimicrobial pretreatment rinse

9. Scale deposits

10. Clean denture

11. Selectively polish

12. Fluoride treatment

Appointment #2 (twenty minutes/two weeks later)

1. Re-evaluate palatal mucosa

2. Take plaque and bleeding index

3. Have client demonstrate home care regimen

4. Re-appoint three months

Summary

Dental hygiene care planning and appointment planning represent the integration of the client's assessment and mutually agreed on health care goals. The care plan identifies the interventions necessary to meet the overall goal or goals and provides a listing of specific outcomes. Following the development of the care plan, the appointment plan is formulated by sequencing and organizing the interventions into an appropriate format. Time elements, clinician's skill level, client's needs, and equipment available determines the length of each appointment and the number of procedures that can be performed. All of this information is presented to the client in the next phase of the dental hygiene process of care, implementation.

REFERENCES

Cacioppo, J., & Petty, R. (1981). Central and peripheral routes to persuasion: The role of message repetition. In L. Alwitt & A. Mitchell (Eds.), *Psychological processes and advertising effects*, Hillsdale: Lawrence-Erlbaum.

Logan, H. (1991). Communication and persuasion: Factors influencing a patient's behavior. *Journal of Dental Education, 55*, 570–574.

Petty, R., & Cacioppo, J. (1981). *Attitudes and persuasion: Classic and contemporary approaches*. Dubuque, IA: William Brown.

Woodall, I. R. (1993). *Comprehensive dental hygiene care* (4th ed.). St. Louis, MO: Mosby-Year Book.

Exercise 5.1 The Parts of an Outcome Statement

Identify the parts—subject (S), performance (P), conditions (CD), and criteria (CR)—of the outcome statements that are provided.

1. Inflammation will be eliminated by the removal of denture for 6 to 8 hours daily.

2. Potential for infection of third molar area will be reduced by the daily use of irrigation.

Exercise 5.2 Planning for Evaluation

For each situation below, what specific type of evaluation would you use and when would you apply it?

1. Eliminate palatal inflammation under denture

2. Reduce plaque by 50 percent

3. Reduce cariogenic food in diet

4. Institute daily use of fluoride

5. Maintain periodontal health without further bone loss

Exercise 5.3 Writing Goal Statements

Write a goal statement for the following dental hygiene diagnosis:

> Localized keratinization of buccal vestibular mucosa related to smokeless tobacco use

List the dental hygiene interventions that would be appropriate.
Establish an appointment plan.

CHAPTER 6

Implementation

Learning Outcomes

At the completion of the chapter the reader should be able to:

1. Describe the procedures required to prepare the operatory and equipment for client treatment
2. Describe strategies of behavior change that promote compliance
3. Describe various formats for recording information in client charts
4. Effectively communicate care plans to the client

INTRODUCTION

Implementation, the fourth phase of the dental hygiene process of care, is the act of putting the dental hygiene care plan into operation. The dental hygiene interventions that are described in the care plan are performed to achieve the care plan's goals and expected outcomes. If not already presented during planning, the implementation phase is the point at which the care plan is presented to the client. Before any specific procedures can be performed, the client should be informed and consent to the planned course of treatment.

However, in practice settings immediate implementation of dental hygiene interventions is sometimes necessary. For instance, when reviewing a client's medical history, the client experiences a medical emergency that requires the dental hygienist to take immediate action. Other situations may arise when assessing the client that would prompt the dental hygienist to implement a specific procedure. For example, a new client presents for an initial assessment and examination. Upon evaluation of the periodontium the dental hygienist finds that the client is extremely sensitive to probing. Therefore, to complete the periodontal assessment accurately, the dental hygienist needs to provide the client with a topical anesthetic agent. Although these circumstances do arise, the implementation phase usually follows the care planning component of the dental hygiene process.

PREPROCESS

At this point, a gap exists between the expertly planned individualized dental hygiene care plan and the implementation of the interventions. Even though the care plan can be tailored to meet the individualized needs of the client, if not communicated effectively, it is doomed to failure. Implementation cannot proceed until the client understands and accepts the planned care (McCullough, 1993). By communicating effectively there is a decrease in client fear, a building of trust, and the formation of a relationship that maximizes positive outcomes.

The terms *case presentation, consultation,* and *informed consent* can be used interchangeably to describe the action of communicating the care plan to the client. Informed consent is the legal reason to avoid litigation and misunderstandings.

The following are some guidelines for presenting the care plan to the client:

1. **State the client's problems in understandable terms.** During the assessment phase the dental hygienist needs to identify the client's educational and maturity level so that appropriate levels of communication can be utilized. It would be inappropriate to speak above the client's educational level—he or she might be too embarrassed to ask questions and just accept the plan without true understanding. On the other hand, speaking below the client's educational level strains your relationship by your not recognizing your client's own expertise and understanding. Media terms and layman's terms should also be used to explain situations. For example, using the term tartar instead of calculus, and infection instead of inflammation may be more understandable. Visual aids, in addition to the client's radiographs, and study models are helpful.

2. **Describe the suggested plan of care.** When describing the care plan, include a discussion of the potential benefits and risks, costs, and time involved. This will minimize surprises and ensure full understanding.

3. **Identify alternative treatment options.** Although the suggested care plan seems to be the best choice from a health care provider's standpoint, it may not meet the needs of the client. Therefore, alternatives allow the client to participate in the decision-making process and choose the most compatible care plan.

Some experts suggest the use of a signed contractual agreement between the health care provider and the client to reduce the possibility of legal actions (Rozovsky, 1990; Pollack, 1987). A contractual agreement, besides providing legal assurance, may act as a client motivator. People who respond well to agreements would be less likely to break scheduled appointments and be motivated to fulfill the contract. In the event that the client refuses the recommended treatment, a treatment refusal letter signed by the client is advised (see Figure 6.1). This will minimize the possibility of legal claims rising from an uninformed client or inappropriate treatment.

In 1973, the American Hospital Association published a bill of rights for the health care consumer. The purpose of the bill was to improve the quality of care

I, _____ , the undersigned, being of lawful age,

hereby release from liability Dr. _____ , and his or her

associates, employees, and agents from any injury I may currently, or in the future

suffer as a result of my refusal to have the following service(s) or consultations(s)

performed:

_____

_____

_____

_____

The need for the services(s) or consultations(s) has been fully explained to me,

along with the consequences of not having the service(s) or consultation(s) per-

formed.

I have discussed the matter with the care provider, all my questions have been

answered, and I fully understand why the recommendation has been made, and

the effects of my refusal.

_____   _____
(Signature of Client)   (Print Name)

_____   _____
(Signature of Client)   (Print Name)

_____   _____
(Signature of Client)   (Print Name)

                                                              _____
                                                                       (Date)

Figure 6.1   *Sample refusal letter*

and increase client satisfaction. Today this bill of rights is posted in most hospital
rooms and medical offices. The American Dental Association and the American
Dental Hygienists' Association, as well as the Commission on Dental Accreditation,
also requires that a written policy on client rights and client access to comprehen-
sive health care be established for both school-based clinics and private offices.
Figure 6.2 is a sample of the clients' bill of rights that was developed for the State
University of New York College of Technology at Farmingdale Dental Hygiene
Care Center. The clients' bill of rights is posted in the reception area to inform

CLIENT'S BILL OF RIGHTS

The students, faculty and staff at the SUNY Farmingdale Dental Hygiene Care Center strive to provide high quality care in a friendly atmosphere. All of our clients are entitled to:

- Considerate and respectful treatment in a clean and safe environment

- Receive treatment without discrimination as to race, color, religion, sex, national origin, disability, sexual orientation, or source of payment

- Continuity and completion of dental hygiene care that meets the professional standard

- Advance knowledge of the cost of the dental hygiene service

- Access to complete and current information about his/her oral conditions

- Receive information that is needed to give informed consent for any proposed procedure or treatment

- An explanation of the recommended dental hygiene treatment, treatment alternatives, and the expected outcome

- Refuse treatment and be told what effect this may have on their oral health

- Confidentiality regarding their medical condition, oral health, and patient records

Figure 6.2   *Client's bill of rights, (Courtesy State University of New York—Farmingdale)*

the public on the institution's statement of clients' rights and access to care. It also appears in the clinic manual and is communicated to all students, faculty, and staff members at the beginning of each semester.

Prior to implementing the dental hygiene care plan the dental hygienist needs to reassess the client's needs, determine if any new data is present and modify the dental hygiene care plan accordingly. As previously mentioned in Chapter 2, the assessment phase is continuous and interacts with other components of the dental hygiene process to ensure that the proposed dental hygiene intervention is appropriate for meeting the client's individual needs and achieving the desired outcomes.

IMPLEMENTATION PROCESS

The implementation process consists of the actions necessary to carry out the dental hygiene plan of care. Preparation of the operatory, performance of the procedures, after care, and recording the treatment rendered are all part of the implementation process.

Preparation

Proper infection control procedures are necessary to reduce the potential for cross contamination in the dental operatory. Hepatitis C and tuberculosis are two specific pathogens that are increasing in prevalence (Kelly, 1993; Yoder, 1993). These pathogens, in addition to the HIV virus and the easily transmitted hepatitis B virus, are just a few of the pathogens that place the health care provider and the client at risk.

Protection of the client and the clinician must be a priority of the dental hygienist. The Center for Disease Control (CDC) and the Occupational Safety and Health Administration (OSHA) have established guidelines and recommendations for the dental office. The American Dental Hygienists' Association (ADHA) along with the American Federation of State, County, and Municipal Employees, the Service Employees International Union, and the American Nurses Association strongly support the OSHA standard for Occupational Exposure to Bloodborne Pathogens. These groups believe that the standard has had a positive impact on the health care industry and substantially increased worker safety and health. ADHA president Sarah A. Turner, RDH, MAE, also stated that the standard "is designed to protect the employees as well as ultimately protect the public we all serve. Safety for the employees and the public remain paramount . . ." (Lyons, 1993).

Infection control procedures involve three distinct areas: personal protective equipment, treatment room sanitization and disinfection, and instrument sterilization. When the proper infection control procedures are performed, the potential for client or clinician contamination is drastically reduced.

Personal protective equipment includes those items that directly protect the clinician, such as gloves, protective eye wear or face shield, mask, and appropriate clinical attire. In addition, immunizations, specifically the hepatitis B vaccination, intact skin, and proper handwashing will help to decrease the potential for contamination. The term "Universal Precautions" is used to remind health professionals to assume that all clients are potential carriers of infectious diseases, including HBV and HIV. In other words, treat everyone the same, don't pick and choose your protective equipment based on how well you know your client or his or her appearance.

Each client is entitled to a properly cleaned and disinfected operatory. Since there is a minimal amount of time allotted for treatment room disinfection, it is useful to classify the items in the operatory into critical, semicritical, and noncritical categories (see Exercise 6.1). The Centers for Disease Control and Prevention (1993) defined each category according to its risk of transmitting infection.

Critical items are those that come in direct contact with the client and are used to penetrate soft tissue, such as probes and scalers. These items must be disposable or sterilizable.

Semicritical items consist of those items that become directly contaminated during treatment but do not penetrate soft tissue, such as mouth mirror, saliva ejectors, prophy angles, and prophy cups, for example. These items should be disposable, or sterilized after each use. If the item is not disposable and cannot be sterilized, the item should receive at a minimum high-level disinfection.

Noncritical items are those items in the operatory that become indirectly contaminated during treatment procedures. Since these items have a low risk of transmitting infection, they may be reprocessed with an intermediate level disinfectant. Some examples would be the light handle, bracket tray handle, light switch, chair buttons, and countertops. Extraneous items in the operatory should be kept to a minimum and those that are present should be routinely cleaned and disinfected. Barrier wrapping these items prior to each treatment appointment will help to reduce the potential for contamination, especially of those items that are difficult to clean.

The environment is another aspect of the dental operatory that should be considered. New products are available to help reduce the use of aerosols in the dental operatory. Some examples are high-speed evacuation and air filtering systems. The airflow systems filter and recirculate clean air into the operatory, thereby reducing cross contamination by airborne pathogens. If you do not have access to an airflow system, make sure that the operatory has proper ventilation and access to fresh air.

Radiographic equipment, x-ray machine buttons, cone, head, and film holder should also be protected from contamination. The semicritical items are the film and the film holder. Once the film has been contaminated, proper aseptic technique should be followed until the contaminated protective wrapping on the film is disposed of properly. The most frequent break in the chain of asepsis is the improper handling of contaminated film packets. Noncritical items that become contaminated during the course of the radiographic procedure include door handles, buttons, cone, and head. These items should be barrier wrapped for easy change between clients, or cleaned and disinfected.

Instrument sterilization should be accomplished by the use of an approved sterilization method. Items should be packaged before sterilization and remain packaged until use. Biological indicators should be routinely employed to ensure that the sterilization method is working properly.

An effective and efficient routine needs to be developed for establishing proper infection control in the practice of dental hygiene. A specific routine will decrease the chance of overlooking contaminated items and greatly decrease the potential for cross contamination.

Other routines that are essential include having instruments and supplies ready and available for client treatment. Gauze and a sharpening stone in an instrument kit reduces the likelihood of cross contamination. Appointment planning requires efficient use of time. Equipment must be readily available and in good working order. Instruments must be sharp and the supply of a sufficient quantity to provide care to a succession of clients who may present with the same characteristics. Support for behavioral interventions includes oral physiotherapy aids and audiovisual resources that support educational efforts. Because our time with the client to impart the essential information is so short, brochures and pamphlets serve as reminders and additional sources of information. The key to the preparation phase is good organization and attention to detail.

Performance

The implementation of performance is providing or assisting in providing services necessary for achieving the expected outcomes identified in the dental hygiene care plan. The actual procedures performed on the client require knowledge of dental hygiene theory, competence in performing manual skills, and an attitude of care and concern for the client. The procedures range from initial therapy and periodontal debridement, to caries control, nutrition counseling, and home care education/instruction, depending on the clients needs.

The most difficult task or procedure the dental hygienist faces is the one that includes client participation. It is easy for the client to be passive and receive treatment, but if the goal is to achieve better oral hygiene and the objective is to have the client perform a daily home care procedure, accomplishing the goal becomes very difficult. Three scenarios can occur: First, the client understands what needs to be done, is motivated and takes it upon him- or herself to accomplish it. Second, the client understands what needs to be done, is not motivated, and is reluctant to perform the procedure. Third, the client does not understand what needs to be done, is not motivated, and will not perform the procedure. Of course the first scenario is the ideal situation—the client assumes responsibility. Unfortunately, the two other scenarios are more common. There are three reasons an individual may not perform positive health behaviors: inadequate knowledge, inadequate skill, or inadequate motivation.

Inadequate knowledge relates directly to the dental hygienist. Client education is an important part of the implementation phase and necessary for successful client participation. Understanding learning theory is helpful when trying to educate your client. The following is a list of statements from Conley (1973), a learning theorist, who identified some learning generalizations.

1. **Learning requires perceiving.** The learner must perceive the situation or subject as important and relevant or needed in order for learning to occur.

2. **Unique characteristics of the learner govern the extent of what is integrated.** Research has consistently proven that learning differences exist among individuals, therefore an explanation that worked for one client may not be appropriate for another.

3. **The degree of learning is influenced by one's environment.** It has been demonstrated that the environment is an important variable affecting learning. For some clients, the dental operatory may be intimidating and decrease the clients learning potential. These clients may need to read some literature at home or have instruction conducted in another type of room in the dental office.

4. **Learning is dependent upon the activity of the learner.** When one has a need or drive to learn, problem solve, or accomplish, one is motivated to satisfy this need.

5. **Motivation of the learner influences what is learned.** Internal motives such as achievement, esteem, and self-actualization as well as external drives and incentives must be considered. Both play an important role in determining what is learned.

6. **Reinforcement of desired behavior increases the probability that the behavior will reoccur in another situation.** Positive reinforcement of specific behaviors has been shown to be effective.

7. Transfer of learning occurs when similar conditions are present in old and new situations. In other words, a stimulus pattern that produces a certain response will tend to replicate the response if it or a similar pattern is repeated. This occurs when learning or the performance of a desired behavior is not carried through at the first appointment. The client was motivated to floss right after the appointment, but after one week the behavior stopped. By replicating the position of "need" at another time, even by another health care provider, the client may continue the desired behavior until it becomes routine.

8. Practice determines the effectiveness and efficiency in learning. Practice periods and evaluation between appointment intervals facilitate learning and decrease the chance of losing the motivation.

Improving a client's skill level may be accomplished by education or by the introduction of a modified oral physiotherapy device. Some clients are not able to brush properly because of poor dexterity related to arthritis. Modification of the toothbrush handle may be all that is necessary to improve their level of skill.

In addition to obtaining knowledge and improving skill, the client needs to be motivated. Motivation may be affected by poor time management. A frequent excuse heard by the dental hygienist from clients is that it takes too much time to perform the tasks required. Helping the client fit the needed performance into his or her schedule may be all that is necessary to have the client implement the new behavior. This is a form of behavior modification that is the key to continued behavior change.

Behavior modification is based on the assumption that behavior is a function of environmental events that precede and follow the behavior. The concept is defined as a chain of events: *antecedent, behavior, consequence,* or *A-B-C.* An antecedent to a behavior could also be described as the stimulus or cue to the behavior. The following are three ways to enhance the stimulus, and hence motivate the client.

1. Design environments to make behavior change convenient or comfortable. An example would be to move dental floss next to the chair by the television so the client can floss while watching the evening news. Once the habit is established the music preceding the news will tend to activate the behavior.

2. Add reminders. A habit can be established by a note on the bathroom mirror, such as "FLOSS!!!", or attached to refrigerator, "NO SWEETS BETWEEN MEALS!!!" Significant others, people important to the client, can be enlisted to help remind.

3. Obtain written commitment. Signing a contract is considered important. Making a promise and keeping it is a matter of pride for many and a serious motivational tool.

The second aspect of behavior modification assesses consequences to behavior, or the BC relationship versus the AC relationship. Consequences of a behavior can be either pleasant/positive, and therefore reinforce the behavior, or unpleasant/negative and act as a punisher. Positive reinforcement strengthens the chance that the behavior will be repeated. However, when a consequence is viewed as unpleasant, once it is removed it is then a strong negative reinforcer. As

an example, the clean, fresh breath feeling following brushing is a positive reinforcer. However, if a person experiences dentinal hypersensitivity each time he or
she brushes, brushing behavior will most likely be limited. Teaching the client
methods to reduce the sensitivity, thus reducing the negative consequence of
brushing, will be negative reinforcement but still affect the behavior in a positive
manner.

There are many ways to reinforce behavior. In Chapter 4 other determinents of
health behavior were discussed. It is necessary to take those distinguishing personality types into consideration prior to designing the specific intervention and motivational approach. Oral health as a concept and its importance to the individual
determines readiness for change to occur. For instance, if pain is an issue, elimination of that consequence is the goal. Depending on the practitioner's or client's
orientation, the human needs model of physiological or safety needs may be
applied, or the health belief model, in which pain may be viewed by the client as a
serious consequence. Since a condition like dentinal hypersensitivity might not be
alleviated by a simple one-time therapeutic intervention by the dental hygienist,
cooperation and possible behavior change by the client will be required.

Reinforcement of behavior can take many forms. Nonmaterial forms can be as
simple as the social rewards of smiles and encouragement. Offices may use "Cavity
Fighter Clubs" or "Plaque Buster Clubs" with polaroid pictures posted. Public
acknowledgment of success is motivational even for adults. Self-reinforcement can
be accomplished by charting behavior. Plaque indices are excellent to motivate
continued behavior change. Having the client graph behavior to see increases or
decreases as appropriate in the desired behavior are important. There are insufficient visual cues to motivate client behavior in dental hygiene. For instance, in
weight loss programs the scale, a mirror, or a loose waistband are all tangible or
visible clues to success. In dental hygiene, it is important to plan for similar bench-
marks. It makes baseline data collection critical to success. The client must also be
taught to recognize the absence of negative symptoms such as no bleeding when
brushing, and/or no more pink toothbrush. Photographs of before and after
treatment and a hand mirror are all tools to help the client assess progress.

Material rewards can also be considered. If saving money is important to the
client, a percentage reduction of the customary fee for a maintenance visit or the
need for less frequent maintenance appointments may be linked to an improved
gingival, periodontal, or plaque index score.

The performance stage of implementation requires the dental hygienist to
remain current in all aspects of health care. Continuing education courses, professional meetings, professional journals, and networking systems all provide mecha-
nisms to maintain good cognitive, interpersonal, and technical skills. Cognitive
knowledge of the principles and steps of specific procedures, technical skills in
positioning the client and manipulating the equipment, and interpersonal skills to
inform and reassure the client are necessary to implement the care plan successfully and provide the best care possible.

After Care

Following treatment procedures the dental hygienist needs to recap the appointment with the client. If there are any prescriptions or instructions that the client

needs to follow, they should be written down and presented to the client. An explanation of the client's next appointment should be made. If the client is on a maintenance program, then an update on the client's improvement and continued treatment plan should be provided. Although these points of care seem obvious, they are important to remember. The client depends on the dental hygienist to direct and follow up care.

Recording

Once the client's appointment is completed, it is necessary to write a brief description of what has transpired. This is usually called the *treatment-rendered entry.* Some offices use the same form for treatment rendered and fee collection. The entry can range from a narrative to a checkoff list containing the procedures performed. It is the only legal document that identifies the actual treatment provided.

As a legal document, the client's treatment record may be entered into court proceedings as evidence for a number of purposes (e.g., accident or injury claims by the client; malpractice charges against health professionals). The client's chart may be the only evidence that competent care was provided. It also serves as a reference point for other health care providers. For instance, if a client is seen by a different dental hygienist for follow-up care, a reference from the treatment-rendered form can clarify past treatment procedures and client responses. Duplication of efforts is minimized and the continuity of care is enhanced.

The treatment-rendered entry has also been termed the progress note and should contain the following information: client's subjective findings; the clinician's objective findings; any medication administered, such as local anesthetic; the procedure performed; complication and/or results observed; the client's reactions; and whether the treatment is complete or incomplete (Woodall, 1993). All progress notes or treatment-rendered entries should be dated and signed by the health care provider. The time of day may also be included as additional information.

There are many different formats used for recording information. The most common is the *DAR format.* The following is a brief description of this type of treatment documentation.

> **D**—The **data** includes the dental hygiene observations of client status. This might include data from the medical history, periodontal exam, and gingival assessment. It includes both subjective and objective data. This section corresponds to the assessment phase of the dental hygiene process of care.

> **A**—**Action** entries include interventions just performed as well as plans for further action. This step corresponds to the planning and implementation phases of the dental hygiene process of care.

> **R**—**Response** entries describe the client's responses to the dental hygiene interventions. The data in this section consists of client measurements and behaviors, many of which will also be recorded on other chart forms. This section corresponds to the evaluation step in the dental hygiene process of care.

Depending on the situation, documentation of each section may not be relevant. For instance, if it was the client's first appointment and treatment was not complete, the response section would contain limited information. The following is a sample treatment rendered/progress note for a relatively healthy client who is being treated at a maintenance appointment; the treatment interval is four months:

> 1/6/94: Client reports that there is sensitivity to hot and cold on the mandibular left side. Updated health history, vital signs, no radiographic evidence of a pathology, gingival recession present teeth #20, #21, generalized gingival inflammation, light subgingival calculus, no significant periodontal changes. Discussed tooth sensitivity as it relates to gingival recession and tooth abrasion. Reviewed the modified Bass toothbrushing method and suggested the use of a desensitizing toothpaste. Applied professional in-office desensitization with dentin block, ultrasonic and hand instrumentation of all teeth, polished remaining stain with Nupro fine grit, applied 1 four-minute acidulated phosphate fluoride treatment. Client has been flossing and using the proxy-brush on a daily basis. Treatment complete, maintenance interval 4 months.   LMJ

Another format for charting is the *SOAP method.* SOAP is an acronym for subjective data, objective data, assessment, and plan. It can also include implementation and evaluation, in which case it would be termed SOAPIE. When using this format, the focus of each component should be on the dental hygiene diagnosis.

S— **Subjective data** is information obtained from what the client expresses. It describes the client's perspectives, perceptions, and experience of the problem. When possible, quote the client's words: otherwise, summarize the statement. Include subjective data only when it is important and relevant to the problem.

O— **Objective data** consists of information that can be measured or observed by use of the senses (e.g., vital signs, probing depths, X-ray results). The objective data section is also used to record interventions that have been carried out (e.g., taught correct flossing technique). Note that this differs from the definition in Chapter 2, which states that data is information about the client. In the SOAP recording method, objective data refers to dental hygiene interventions as well as client responses.

A— The **assessment** is an interpretation or explanation of the subjective and objective data. Following the initial assessment, the dental hygiene diagnosis is formulated and should be stated in this section. The assessment should also describe the client's condition and level of progress.

P— The **plan** is the plan of care designed to resolve the stated problem. Its focus is on specific dental hygiene interventions that will restore or maintain oral health.

I— **Intervention** is a description of the actual procedures that were performed or instructions that were given.

E— The **evaluation** describes the results of treatment and success of the plan.

The following is a case entry using the SOAPIE format.

1/20/94:

S— Client stated, "My gums bleed every time I floss."

O— Medical history unremarkable, enlarged interproximal papilla, floss cuts surrounding papilla, moderate amounts of interproximal plaque.

A— Inflammed interproximal gingival tissues related to knowledge and skill deficit concerning the usage of dental floss. Client ineffectively using dental floss by evidence of floss cuts and presence of interproximal plaque.

P— Instruct on proper floss procedure, remove supra- and subgingival deposits.

I— Gave floss instruction via demonstration on typodont and client. Observed client's usage and gave feedback. Scaled remaining areas of plaque accumulation.

E— States understanding of flossing procedure, is motivated to continue to floss on a daily basis. Reevaluate 3 months.

LJM

Chart entries can be shortened by using abbreviations as long as the abbreviations are well known and can be easily interpreted. It is important to remember that all entries should be complete, accurate, legible, with the author easily identified, and in ink or some other permanent form (Pollack, 1987). Never skip a line—if the entry does not fill the entire writing space, draw a line to the margin and sign. Records can be easily altered if space is left between entries. When errors are made in an entry, a single line should be drawn through it, the word "error" written above it, and the correction made on the next available line (Pollack, 1987). It is also a good policy to initial any such changes.

In addition to chart entry formats there are three types of systems of record-keeping utilized in the documentation of client care. They are (1) source-oriented records, (2) problem-oriented records, and (3) computer-assisted records.

The *source-oriented record system* is the traditional charting system; it continues to be utilized by a number of institutions and agencies and in many private dental offices. In this system, information is recorded chronologically within specific time periods. When used in a multidisciplinary setting such as a hospital or nursing home, the medical record is divided into sections according to the source of the data. Each discipline records information in a separate section—for example, dental notes, physical therapy notes, nurses' notes, and physician notes.

The *problem-oriented record system* of documentation parallels the process of care. It involves data collection, identification of client problems (diagnoses), development and implementation of the plan of care, and evaluation of outcome achievement. In this system, information focuses on the client's problems (diagnoses) and integrates all disciplines by utilizing a consistent format. All health professionals, regardless of discipline, record on the same forms. The entire team contributes to a master list of client problems and to the plan of care for each problem. The following are the basic components of the problem-oriented record.

1. Defined database. The database consists of all the initial information about the client's health: personal profile, history, physical examination findings, and diagnostic studies.

2. Master problem list. The initial problem list is developed from the database. All health care professionals contribute to the problem list, which may contain medical, dental, psychological, sociocultural, and spiritual problems. Problems are listed in the order in which they are identified and the list is usually found at the front of the chart. Figure 6.3 is a sample of the problem list form used at the Veterans Administration Hospital in Northport, New York.

3. Problem-oriented plan of care. An initial plan is developed for each problem on the master list. Dentists write plans for dental problems, dental hygienists write plans for dental hygiene problems, physicians write plans for medical problems. Note that in this system the care plan is not a separate document, but is integrated within the progress notes in the client's chart.

4. Multidisciplinary progress notes. In this section, all health professionals involved in the client's care make narrative entries that correspond to the problems on the master list.

The problem-oriented system of charting is beneficial in the sense of developing collaborative relationships between health care professionals. It also facilitates the tracking of an individual problem and improves the awareness of treatments performed by other members of the health care team.

Computer-assisted records are slowly becoming a part of the dental practice. They have the advantage of sorting and cross referencing data, providing financial management of the client's account, and minimizing the potential for cross contamination when documenting assessment or treatment information. The systems that are available can be tailored to meet the needs of the office or institution. Depending on the type of information to be stored in a computer file, computer terminals may be located in the dental operatory, reception area, and/or financial office.

Summary

The implementation phase of dental hygiene process of care contains the actual actions that put the dental hygiene care plan into operation. It is composed of case presentation, reassessment, preparation, performance, after care, and recording. Each step is vital to the success of treatment. As the dental hygiene process of care unfolds, it is easy to see how all phases are interdependent.

MEDICAL RECORD	PROBLEM LIST	*(Check one)* ☐ FIRST LIST *(New)*　　☐ CONTINUATION OF LIST

DO NOT USE ABBREVIATIONS WHEN LISTING PROBLEMS. This form may be used for inpatient, patient – members and outpatients. Place form in the Medical Records folder (Type II) on the top of right or left side, whichever is appropiate. Upon READMISSION, remove form and place with current records on ward. DO NOT CREATE A NEW Problem List for each readmission.

PROBLEM NUMBER	APPROX. DATE OF ONSET	DATE PROBLEM RECORDED	ACTIVE PROBLEMS	INACTIVE/RESOLVED *(Add date)*

ENTER IN SPACE BELOW: PATIENT IDENTIFICATION –TREATMENT FACILITY – WARD NO. – DATE

(CONTINUE ON REVERSE)

MEDICAL RECORD

PROBLEM LIST

VA FORM 10-1415
APRIl 1976

EXISTING STOCK OF VA FORM 10-1415
MAY 1974, WILL BE USED.

Figure 6.3　*Sample problem list, Northport Veterans Hospital, NY*

REFERENCES

Centers for disease control and prevention (1993). Recommended infection control practice for dentistry. *Access,* (Sept.) pp. 48–52.

Conley, B. (1973). *Curriculum and instruction in nursing* (pp. 212–214). Boston: Little & Brown.

Kelly, M. (1993, March). Tuberculosis and hepatitis C. *Practical Hygiene,* p. 32.

Lyons, S. (1993, December). Whatever OSHA says, goes and stays. *Access, 7,* 19.

McCullough, C. (1993, May). Case presentation/effective communication. *Access, 10,* 37–39.

Pollack, B. (1987). *Handbook of dental jurisprudence and risk management.* Littleton, MA: PSG Publishing.

Rozovsky, F. (1990). *Consent to treatment: Practical guide.* Boston: Little & Brown.

Woodall, I. (1993). *Comprehensive dental hygiene care.* 4th ed. St. Louis, MO: Mosby-Year Book Inc.

Yoder, K. (1993, May). Tuberculosis: A re-emerging hazard for oral health care workers. *Journal of Dental Hygiene, 67,* 208.

Exercise 6.1   Infection Control

Identify the following items as critical, semicritical, and noncritical in terms of infection control.

1. suction tips   _____

2. operator chair   _____

3. instructional material   _____

4. light handle   _____

5. film packet   _____

6. dental explorer   _____

7. picture on wall   _____

8. pens used for charting   _____

9. client bib   _____

10. fluoride tray   _____

Exercise 6.2   Problem Solving

When educating a client who understands or perceives the situation as a problem but does not follow through with instructions, the situation is one of:

Behavior modification through motivation   OR
Learning style difficulty

Identify three ways in which the problem can be solved.

_____

_____

_____

_____

CHAPTER 7

Evaluation of Dental Hygiene Care

Learning Outcomes

At the completion of the chapter the reader should be able to:

1. Identify the universal characteristics of evaluation
2. Describe the three types of evaluation
3. Discuss the evaluation methods used to determine client progress toward outcome achievement
4. Choose the correct method of evaluation to assess client health status
5. Define the terms beneficence and maleficence
6. Analyze the structure, process, and outcome of clinical practice and programs to assure quality

INTRODUCTION

Although evaluation may be last in the list of the elements of the dental hygiene process, it should not be viewed as the final step. Evaluation is rooted in the assessment phase that provided the baseline data that will be the foundation of the evaluation. Formulation of the evaluation component continues during the diagnosis and planning as outcome identification. Evaluation is built into the implementation phase of the care plan to monitor progress of therapies and interventions. Finally, evaluation itself leads to reassessment and revised or redesigned care plans.

UNIVERSAL CHARACTERISTICS OF EVALUATION

Formal evaluation is a systematic process by which a judgment is made about a *value, worth,* or *quality* of something by comparing it to a *previously identified set of criteria or standards.* A *standard* is established by authority. It is a consensus or model of something that has quality or value. Dental hygiene standards are based on scientific and ethical knowledge and currently accepted practice. They may be used to judge clinical performance, for instance. Mostly they are broad and require criteria to make judgments. *Criteria* are measurable and observable qualities. They are the tools by which standards can be measured. The American Academy of Periodontology defines periodontal health by certain defining characteristics or parameters of probe depth, mobility, attachment loss, and so forth that set a standard. The various indices and measurements used to determine periodontal health status are evaluation tools. The criteria are the desired outcomes by using the evaluative tools such as <3 mm attachment loss or 75 percent plaque reduction on a Navy Plaque Index.

The important thing to remember is that criteria must be established in conjunction with the original goal. If the goal of the care plan is "reduced decay," then a bleeding on probing index would be an inappropriate evaluative tool. Although this may seem ridiculously simple, clinicians may frequently use inappropriate indices to measure a program's results or misread the importance of the results. A criteria or index must be *valid* and *reliable.* Validity of a measure means it measures what it is intended to measure. A plaque index is a good example. A low plaque score means there is no plaque present at the time of the measurement. It does not measure gingival health, periodontal health, or the client's skill in plaque removal over a period of time. Alone, all it tells us is that the client effectively removed plaque prior to the application of the index by any means at his or her disposal. Used alone, it is not valid to judge anything else. To make any judgment, additional criteria such as bleeding on probing, or gingival or periodontal indices must be used to meet the standard of periodontal health.

Criteria must also be reliable. That means it yields the same results each time. Each index used in dentistry has a set of rules. When the clinician records an Oral Hygiene Index (OHI) of 3.2, that should immediately conjure a picture of the client's condition to all who are familiar with the index. Similarly, certain readings—such as blood pressure or temperature, observable scores of respiration, or probe readings—all fall within preset standards or parameters that determine "health," or least acceptable degrees of health.

TYPES OF EVALUATION

There are three types of evaluation. Two types focus on the individuals involved, namely the clinician and the client, and are termed *process evaluation* and *outcome evaluation.* The third type is *structural evaluation* and draws conclusions regarding the setting in which the interventions occur.

Process evaluation focuses on the activities of the caregiver. It should answer the following questions:

> Is the care relevant to the client's needs?
>
> Is the care appropriate, timely, and complete?

Does the care meet accepted quality standards?

In what manner is the care given?

The care given to the client must be judged to some degree on the clinician's skills. Incomplete removal of calculus, for example, may compromise the desired outcome. Care given in a haphazard ineffective manner may interfere with the resolution of conditions. Clinicians who are rough in handling instruments or brusque in their interpersonal exchanges may not get the needed client cooperation or trust.

Outcome evaluation focuses on the client's health status, satisfaction with therapy, and progress toward goals. It evaluates how the intervening therapy contributes to goal achievement. It should answer the questions:

To what degree were the client's goals achieved?

To what degree did the intervention contribute?

The third type of evaluation, structural, directs attention to the setting in which the intervention takes place. It may evaluate the office setting in terms of appointment planning, organization, or qualifications of personnel:

Is there sufficient time and resources to provide quality care?

Are the skills of personnel providing or supporting the provision
of therapy appropriate to the tasks?

Structural evaluation may also look at aspects that specifically refer to the client's surroundings. For the nonambulatory or disabled, this is a critical question. The client's community resources should also be considered. Knowing where to buy essential oral care products you recommend can promote goal achievement. For example, the client frustrated because he or she is unable to find a replacement proxibrush may not comply with your recommendations.

The ultimate goal of evaluation is to determine the client's progress toward goal achievement, and determine the effectiveness of the dental hygiene care plan. To be effective, the universal requisites must be to determine quality or value and to use preselected criteria or standards.

The time that data is collected is essential to evaluation. One cannot judge the degree to which a problem has been resolved if there is no baseline data with which to compare. Data collected in the assessment phase becomes the benchmark by which we compare the outcome at future appointments. The purpose in the assessment phase was to aid in diagnosis. The same evaluation tool must be used at future appointments to enable accurate comparisons. It would be invalid, for instance, to use two different gingival indices. Even though both are measuring the same condition, comparison would be difficult. Evaluation data enables a judgment to be made about any change in the client's oral health status (Table 7.1). If the evaluation data are collected throughout a series of appointments, as in process evaluation, the results help to direct the further course of treatment.

Table 7.1 • TIME AND PURPOSE OF DATA COLLECTION		
	Assessment Data	Evaluation
When collected	In assessment phase before care is given	In evaluation phase after care is given
Purpose	Diagnosis of client status	Evaluation of change in client status

METHODS OF EVALUATION

There are three ways to gather data for evaluation. The first is *direct observation* of the client by the clinician. Second is *examination of the chart.* The client may have been seen by other dental team members, thus chart entries may have a direct bearing on the evaluation. Lastly, a *client interview* enables the clinician to evaluate progress to the outcome by the client's responses.

The methods of evaluation can be applied to each of five aspects of the client's health status, namely, function and appearance, specific symptoms, knowledge, psychomotor skills, and attitude. While all three methods may be applied to each aspect some will have more value than others as indicated below.

Function and Appearance—Function includes general appearance of the client and oral cavity as well as the functional aspect of the oral cavity. The data gathered is compared to that of the initial assessment to evaluate progress toward the desired outcome. Examples: Appearance may include amount of stain, appearance of teeth and smile, or halitosis. Function would evaluate intact mucosa, tooth mobility, and ability to chew and swallow. Evaluation methods of choice: All three methods of evaluation have value and will contribute information.

Specific Symptoms—All the signs and symptoms of actual or potential disease need to be evaluated for the degree that they have been resolved. Examples: Bleeding on probing, probe depth, decalcification, suppuration, lymphadenopathy, and the frequency and duration of symptom occurrence such as pain. Evaluation methods of choice: All three methods may have value, but direct observation and client interview will most likely yield the best information.

Knowledge—The client's knowledge of symptoms that signal the disease process, disease etiology, preventive measures, complications of ignoring symptoms, or not using preventive measures have a direct impact on ability to achieve the desired outcome. Examples: Recall of previously given information, comprehension, and application are all to be evaluated. Evaluation method of choice: Client interview is the most efficient method.

Psychomotor Skills—Ability to perform the function taught is necessary to achieve the goals. Example: Are alterations necessary to the oral physiotherapy aids or is additional training required? Evaluation methods of choice: Direct observation is necessary.

Attitude—Incorporation of a new behavior into one's lifestyle is largely dependent on attitude. Skill and knowledge may be a prerequisite, but do not in and of themselves assure success. Examples: Evaluate the congruency of signs and symptoms with the reported behavior. Encourage open sharing of feelings and attitudes toward therapy and to preventive maintenance or other changes. Evaluation methods of choice: Client interview as well as direct observation are the methods of choice to ascertain the information.

EVALUATION OF CLIENT PROGRESS

Since the purpose of evaluation is to judge the degree to which a client has progressed to the health status goal, the dental hygienist must make judgments about the *actual outcome*, which is the client's response to the *predicted outcome* stated in the planning step. The evaluation may be *ongoing* throughout the course of treatment, as in taking a plaque score at each appointment, or *terminal* at the end of the series of appointments, as exemplified by a full mouth probing one month following initial periodontal debridement.

The professional standards of the American Dental Hygienists' Association (1985) identify evaluation of dental hygiene therapy as the responsibility of the dental hygienist. Performance evaluation procedures assure the intervention instituted by the hygienist has actually met the client's needs. Without evaluation, therapy becomes a rote set of procedures that may constitute overtreatment, undertreatment, or inappropriate treatment. Only by evaluating the client's progress in relation to the care plan can the dental hygienist know whether to continue, change, or terminate therapy.

Finally, by identifying specific dental hygiene interventions that improve client health status, evaluation demonstrates to both employer and consumer the role the dental hygienist plays in achieving client health. Evaluation enables the dental hygienist to improve care by efficiently removing unsuccessful interventions and replacing them with effective therapies.

For each of the client's dental hygiene diagnoses the clinician should

1. review the stated goals or predicted outcomes;
2. collect data about the client's responses to dental hygiene interventions;
3. compare actual outcomes to predicted outcomes and make judgments about whether the goals were met; and
4. record the evaluative statements.

Review Predicted Outcomes—The predicted outcomes were identified in the planning stage. They described how the client would look, do, or feel following dental hygiene interventions.

Collect Evaluation Data—Referencing the dental hygiene diagnosis and the list of predicted outcomes, the dental hygienist uses the three methods of evaluation—direct observation, chart review, and client interview—to collect data. The nature of the goal determines the information. One may question the client about recall of information or have him or her demonstrate a skill.

Compare Actual and Predicted Outcomes and Draw a Conclusion—Three responses are possible. The outcome may be achieved, thus the objective was met. The outcome may be partially achieved, meaning the predicted outcome is met only part of the time. The outcome was not achieved by the target time or the actual outcome didn't meet the predicted outcome. Each type of response needs to be documented and a conclusion drawn. The conclusion drawn is the evaluation.

Outcome Has Been Achieved

The fact that the outcome has been achieved does not necessarily mean that dental hygiene interventions are no longer needed. There are a number of possibilities for additional treatment considerations.

PROBLEM RESOLVED

If the problem is resolved, there is no need for further interventions. This is, of course, the desired outcome. The client complied with the treatment regimen and the clinical interventions were appropriate and effective.

POTENTIAL PROBLEM PREVENTED, RISK FACTORS REMAIN

As long as risk factors remain, the client needs dental/dental hygiene intervention. The care plan may continue as is or be revised to include periodic maintenance and re-evaluation. An example is one in which the dental hygiene diagnosis reads "Knowledge deficit related to improper removal of food under pontic and potential for caries related to pontic device." The outcome addressed incorporation of daily pontic cleansing using a bridge threader into the client's already existing flossing routine. Subsequent evaluation reveals the client is performing the new behavior adequately, however, the pontic traps food and the risk factor for decay of the abutment tooth is still present. Bridge reconstruction is one alternative, shifting treatment to a dental intervention. In this case, the client states that at this time she cannot afford a new bridge. Alternative interventions may include more frequent recalls for evaluation and professionally applied fluoride and/or a regimen of self-applied fluoride delivered to the area of concern with Superfloss or an irrigator.

ACTUAL PROBLEM STILL EXISTS

An example would be a case of toothbrush abrasion. The goal of having the client use a soft bristle toothbrush and appropriate technique were accomplished, however, the abrasion cannot be resolved. The condition can be accepted as not being any threat if no additional symptoms occur or the client can be referred for dental intervention.

Outcome Partially Achieved

Problem reduced, care plan needs revision. The dental hygiene diagnosis for this example was "Plaque accumulation due to limited dexterity." The outcome was to reduce the plaque score by 50 percent in one week using a toothbrush with a bent handle and a floss holder. At the following appointment, the client had a reduced plaque score of only 25 percent. It is obvious the client is still having some dexterity problems, and although he indicated he is still trying hard, plaque is very evident on the lingual surfaces of all the molars. Possibilities for revision could call for additional training, changing the grip of the toothbrush handle, or perhaps the addition of an electric toothbrush.

Problem reduced, continue plan, but allow more time. In this case let's assume the problem was related to smoking. The client was motivated to start a smoking cessation program your office administers. The care plan targeted total cessation in six weeks which ultimately did not occur. The client is still motivated but was unable to meet the expected outcome. Revising the plan needs to address not only an overall timeframe, but perhaps set daily or weekly objectives that are short-term achievable, allowing the client to feel successful.

Outcome Not Achieved

Problem still exists, revise care plan. Not meeting an expected outcome may mean that it was inappropriate because it did not correctly identify the etiology, or the client did not fully comply or agree to the plan. A case in point would be a periodontally involved client who does not heal well or respond to treatment after careful and thorough debridement and other dental hygiene therapy. Among the many options at this point is a reassessment that may include additional dental or medical diagnostic testing of any medical conditions that may be impacting on wound healing, specifying microorganisms for possible antibiotic coverage, and/or additional consultation with the dentist or periodontist, followed by a revision of the dental hygiene care plan as needed.

Problem still exists, continue with care plan of interventions as appropriate. If all evaluations seem to point to the appropriateness of the interventions and expected outcome, as may be the case in many chronic periodontal conditions, the client may remain on a maintenance program. This would be especially true in case of a noncompliant client. The dental hygiene clinical interventions are appropriate and the client will accept frequent recall, but will not make adequate changes in self-care behavior.

Evaluation Errors

The checklists provided in Tables 7.2 to 7.6 will assist the clinician to address each successive step in the dental hygiene process in a systematic manner. In assembling the data, the dental hygienist created a dental hygiene diagnosis that directed the treatment goals, planned interventions, expected outcomes, and the timeframes in which each would be completed and evaluated. Probably the most common evaluation error would be failure to perform the evaluation in a systematic fashion. In a busy office where the emphasis is put on action-oriented treatment rather than analytical procedures, it would be very easy to skip this phase completely. As in all tasks when first learned, they seem to take forever to perform. Many students feel procedures learned in school are really never put into practice. On the contrary, hygienists practicing high-quality care using current concepts use all parts of the dental hygiene process. They may, however, be doing so in a more informal way. As one gains practice in evaluation, for instance, one wouldn't stand with the five evaluation checklists in hand laboriously thinking through each. Rather the practicing hygienist does a mental calculation that may only take a moment or two. The important word to remember is *systematic.* That means the manner in which you review a case is the most important factor. Following assessment, the problem was identified, and should have been written down in the chart as a dental hygiene diagnosis.

Table 7.2 • EVALUATION CHECKLIST—DIAGNOSIS STEP

Questions to ask	Actions to take
1. Is the diagnosis inaccurate or not related to the data?	*Yes. Revise diagnosis.
2. Has the status of the problem changed (actual, possible, potential)?	*Yes. Relabel the problem.
3. Have the factors of etiology and risk been incorrectly reflected?	*Yes. Revise the etiology and/or risk factors.
4. Is the problem one that cannot be treated primarily by independent actions?	*Yes. Consult appropriate health care professional.
5. Is the diagnosis too broad or general (rather than individualized for this client)?	*Yes. Revise diagnosis. Revise goals and care plan as determined by new diagnosis.

Proceed to review the care plan goals.

Table 7.3 • EVALUATION CHECKLIST—CARE PLAN GOALS

Questions to ask	Actions to take
1. Have dental hygiene diagnoses been added or revised?	*Yes. Write new goals.
2. Are there aspects of the client's problem that the goals do not address?	*Yes. Write additional goals.

Proceed to review of the care plan.

Table 7.4 • EVALUATION CHECKLIST—CARE PLAN

Questions to ask	Actions to take
1. Have the dental hygiene diagnosis or goals been added or revised in the previous evaluation steps?	*Yes. Write new care plan.
2. Does the care plan seem unrelated to the client's expectations?	*Yes. Revise or develop new care plan.
3. Does the care plan lack instructions for timing of the interventions?	*Yes. Revise care plan. Add times.
4. Was the intervention(s) ineffective?	*Yes. Delete it.
5. Do the intervention(s) fail to address all aspects of the care plan goals?	*Yes. Revise care plan. Add new interventions.

Proceed to review implementation.

Table 7.5 • **EVALUATION CHECKLIST—IMPLEMENTATION**

Questions to ask	Actions to take
1. Did the dental hygienist fail to get client input at each step in developing and implementing the plan?	*Yes. Obtain client input, revise plan and implementation as needed.
2. Were the dental hygiene interventions unacceptable to the client?	*Yes. Consult client; change interventions or implementation approach.
3. Did the client fail to comply with the therapeutic regimen?	*Yes. Reassess motivation and knowledge. Add goals aimed at teaching, motivating, and supporting change. Set time for re-evaluation.

Proceed to review expected outcomes.

Table 7.6 • **EVALUATION CHECKLIST—EXPECTED OUTCOMES**

Questions to ask	Actions to take
1. Is the outcome unrealistic in terms of the client's abilities or resources?	*Yes. Revise expected outcome.
2. Was sufficient time allowed for outcome achievement?	*Yes. Revise timeframe.
3. Do predicted outcomes fail to demonstrate resolution of the problem specified in the dental hygiene diagnosis?	*Yes. Revise predicted outcomes?
4. Have the client's priorities changed?	*Yes. Revise outcomes and/or care plan.
5. Were they the dental hygienist's objectives rather than the client's?	*Yes. Seek client input. Write outcomes valued by client.

Evaluation complete.

Next, the goals need to be established. If there is one place that a dental hygiene care plan can go wrong, it is probably at this stage. This is so due to communication with the client. Whether the interventions are behavioral or clinical, client cooperation is essential. Care plan interventions are formulated next. Clients are too often overtreated or undertreated. We need to base treatment decisions on sound scientific knowledge and observable clinical data. Remember that quality care is not based solely on delivering the most up-to-date care. It must be based also on how well the care meets the client's needs. The dental hygiene interventions, therefore, will direct the expected outcomes. If interventions are clinical, as quadrant root planing would be, the expected or predicted outcome would be no bleeding on probing at a subsequent visit. If the actual outcome does not meet this objective, the dental hygienist would evaluate at that time why the outcome did not occur. Possibilities of incomplete calculus removal, poor wound healing, active pathogenic process, or inadequate home care would be reviewed and corrections made.

QUALITY ASSURANCE

Quality of health care can be measured by a number of aspects. Since the term quality connotes excellence, there is a degree of subjectivity to the interpretation of its meaning. What is excellent to one may be only adequate to another. Burt and Eklund (1992) further define *quality assessment* as a "measure of quality of care provided in a particular setting." They make the important distinction that *quality assurance* goes beyond assessment or measurement of care and must include "implementation of any necessary changes to either maintain or improve the quality of care rendered." The essential question remains: What constitutes quality?

We must look to professional associations, research, and scientific knowledge, as well as legislation, to direct our determinants. Standards of care can address many varied aspects, such as appropriateness and timeliness of care, documentation, adherence to protocols, oral health status of the client, and outcome of client care. Client satisfaction can also be used to measure quality. It is, however, a somewhat subjective measure, since some studies indicate that since the client cannot accurately judge the quality of the professional's technical skills he or she tends to make the assessment of quality based on the professional's interpersonal skills (Ingersoll, 1982). Costs of care are a further issue of quality. As third party payers, including both insurance companies and government agencies, have more direct impact on private dental practice, the pressure for cost effectiveness and containment increases.

Burt and Eklund (1992) state "if an amalgam restoration could have been avoided through the timely use of fluoride or a sealant, it is hard to think of it as being high quality, even if it has ideal margins and anatomical form." As cost-containment has become a national issue in health care reform, it must become a central issue in any quality assurance program. That does not imply that providing the least expensive treatment is the best, but rather that the most *efficacious* treatment is that of choice. That further translates to preventive treatment over rehabilitative. While the initial cost of a sealant may not be dramatically less than a one surface amalgam, the future costs of replacement restorations and other sequelae must be taken into account. This places the dental hygienist in a critical position. Careful assessment reveals disease in its incipient or prepathologic stage. Initial or preventive therapy is far less costly in both time and dollars.

There are also ethical considerations in quality assurance. In all codes of ethics, there are certain universal moral principles. They include respect for others, confidentiality, veracity, justice, and honesty. They also include or imply the goals *benefi-*

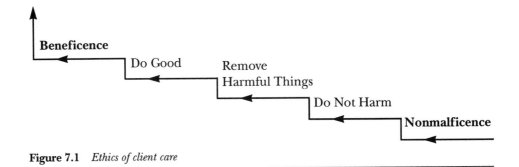

Figure 7.1 *Ethics of client care*

cence, which means doing good, and *nonmalficence*, which means avoiding harm. The range from not harming the individual proceeds along a continuum of trying to prevent harm, to removing things that may be harmful, to finally doing good (Figure 7.1).

Avoiding harm, for instance, means choosing the appropriate care that is preventive, such as a sealant rather than a restoration. Removing harmful things could include thorough root planing that will promote healing. A partial or gross scaling that promotes the formation of a periodontal abscess constitutes maleficence since the partial treatment did more harm than good. An office protocol that dictates gross full mouth ultrasonic scaling at one appointment and quadrant manual scaling at future appointments is an unacceptable sequence of treatment, since it may be increasing the client's risk of abscess rather than reducing it.

An implicit factor in quality assurance is *accountability*, which means being responsible for care activities and being answerable to the client for the activities performed. As licensed professionals, dental hygienists must accept the fact that they have the legal responsibility to direct the dental hygiene portion of client care. No degree of dental supervision in practice acts can supersede that accountability. Education and licensure granted certain rights and concomitant responsibilities.

The American Dental Hygienists' Association's Code of Ethics for Dental Hygienists has been revised and only the first draft was available at the time of this writing. It will be acted upon in the 1995 Annual Session of the Association, with final the form expected after that date (Gaston, 1994).

The draft states that it

> serves a regulatory purpose by establishing a concise benchmark to guide the public's expectations of our profession. It supports existing and future dental hygiene practice, laws, and regulations by providing a foundation for peer review systems and quality assurance measures. By holding ourselves accountable to living up to the standards in the code, we enhance the public's trust on which our professional privilege and status are founded (Gaston, 1994).

The code continues to expand upon several basic beliefs, which include that "we are individually responsible for our actions and the quality of care we provide to our clients" and that "our education and licensure as healthcare professionals qualify us to serve the public by preventing and treating oral disease and helping the public achieve and maintain good health."

The standards of professional responsibility upon which the code is based is multifaceted. It includes colleagues as well as clients, family and friends, and society as a whole. In acknowledging our responsibility to clients, the code delineates the following standards:

1. Provide oral health care utilizing the highest level of professional knowledge, judgment, and skill

2. Maintain a work environment that minimizes the risk of harm to our clients

3. Serve all clients without discrimination

4. Hold professional/client relationships in confidence

5. Communicate with clients in a respectful manner

6. Take action to promote ethical behavior and high standards of care by dental hygienists

7. Serve a client advocate, without regard to personal gain

8. Provide clients with the information necessary to make informed decisions about their oral health

9. Refer the client when his or her needs are beyond our ability or scope of practice

10. Act to educate clients regarding high quality oral health care

EVALUATION FOR QUALITY ASSURANCE

There are several models that have been used to evaluate health care, but the best suited to private practice is Donabedian's (1982). His model uses the methods of structure, process and outcome as previously described. Others have also applied this model to dental practice (Morris, Bentley, Vito, and Bomba, 1988; Schoen, Freed, Gershen, and Marcus, 1989). The components of the model are shown in Table 7.7 and described in the following section.

Table 7.7 • **BASIC PRINCIPLES OF QUALITY ASSESSMENT**

Quality Can Be Inferred from Three Aspects:

Structure	Process	Outcome
Facilities	Elements of performance of care	Effects of care on outcome
Equipment	Chart review	Client satisfaction
Personnel	Dental hygiene process components	Oral hygiene status
Administration	Choice of therapies	Recall frequency

Structure Evaluation

The major assumption relating to structure evaluation is if the organizational structure is optimal, then better quality care will be delivered. There are four elements of structure evaluation: facilities, equipment, personnel and administration.

Facilities—Both the setting and office layout could be evaluated. An important aspect is access. This encompasses access for the handicapped, adequate parking, or access to public transportation and, visible signs identifying the location of the office. It also includes amenities. Is the reception area pleasant, are restroom facilities adequate and operatories conducive to client comfort?

Equipment—In addition to the dental unit and cabinets, instruments and supplies need to be evaluated. Sterilization and storage of sterile supplies should be assessed.

Personnel—This is differentiated from the process evaluation of the caregiver in that this element reviews the appropriateness of the personnel as to sufficient numbers, proper certification and licensure, as well as level of performance. Support of continuing education should be considered as a means of maintaining or improving quality care.

Administration—This is an all-encompassing term that in this instance should be seen in its verb form. What are the procedures, protocols, or rules? How one follows them is the focus of the review. The *record system* is a major issue in this area. Good documentation is critical to quality assurance and therefore the type of chart, its format, and storage are all components to be assessed.

Process Evaluation

Underlying this aspect of evaluation is the assumption that properly managed care leads to good outcomes. Five separate factors to address are case management, records, diagnosis, care plan, and treatment.

Case Management—How a client's case is managed includes having appropriate personnel perform care and the process by which they determine care.

Records—This assesses the specifics of recordkeeping, the completeness and legibility of the entries, and if all the interventions and the client's responses to them have been documented.

Diagnosis—Was the diagnosis appropriate and documented?

Care Plan—Is the plan written; was it sequenced properly?

Treatment—Was the treatment appropriate and timely?

Outcome Evaluation

The general assumption of this component is that health care interventions will change a person's health status. One looks at four categories of outcome evaluation: client satisfaction, oral health status, completion of treatment, and recall pattern.

> **Client Satisfaction**—Interpersonal skills are an important aspect of this factor. Clients who are informed and consent to treatment that they have helped to plan are most likely to be satisfied.
>
> **Oral Health Status**—Each treatment intervention needs to be evaluated in the areas of oral hygiene, tooth loss, periodontal, and caries status.
>
> **Completion of Treatment**—Timeframes of treatment built into the care plan aid in the assessment of timeliness. Careful assessment that identifies early onset of disease is another factor. Completion of treatment is final, meaning the goal or goals were met. If the goal is only partially met, then treatment cannot be considered complete. Therefore, goal formulation is the foundation of this aspect.
>
> **Maintenance Pattern**—The frequency of maintenance needs to be individualized to client need. The client's needs at maintenance are an assessment tool for evaluation. Reduced health status indicates either self-care deficits that need to be addressed or indicate faults in the process, which did not adequately identify the disease, its etiology, or risk factors or apply interventions appropriately.

Criteria and Standards for Quality Assurance Evaluation

When embarking upon a quality assurance review, using the format just described will help to direct the process. Professional associations such as the American Dental Hygienists' Association and the American Dental Association have created Standards of Care that provide additional guidelines for judging quality. Office staff meetings and some brainstorming can identify some areas of concern. Chart audits and client satisfaction surveys are fairly simple methods to initiate a review.

To effect a quality assurance program, standards must be measured using techniques that are valid and reliable. Developing a checklist and applying accepted criteria or protocols of treatments are additional methods. Sometimes working a backwards approach is effective—Start with the desired end result and work backwards, identifying what would have to be accomplished to reach the desired outcome.

Reviewing charts for completeness, either randomly selected or in a systematic pattern, can identify problem areas. Asking the question "If the client requested copies of this chart to be forwarded to another dental practice or initiated a lawsuit tomorrow, would this chart be adequate?" It is not legal to go back and add things to a chart later. Chart entries should be legible and in black pen, no lines skipped and no erasures. Radiographs should be of diagnostic quality including those from previous years. Good radiographic technique, both when exposing and processing films, is important. Improper fixing and rinsing are frequent causes of staining producing poor diagnostic quality when films are viewed at subsequent dates. Recording advice told to the client, such as the dental hygiene diagnosis or the recommended referral to a specialist when necessary, is critical documentation. Chart audits can be a simple way to identify potential problems created by poor documentation. Both the process and outcome evaluation of client care can be judged via an audit.

Clients can be questioned at the end of treatment, formally or informally, to establish the level of satisfaction with the dental hygiene appointments. The clinician or another staff member can ask a few questions at the completion of treatment to judge satisfaction with outcome. Client responses can be recorded in the chart. A short questionnaire may help to give the client a feeling of control and enable him or her to make statements, either positive or negative, that the same client might be reluctant to make verbally.

Summary

Once the review process is complete, one should identify the strengths and weaknesses of the care provided. Specific courses of action need to be chosen to address the weaknesses and correct them. As in all program planning, one would put the identified shortcomings in priority order with the most serious addressed first and each with a timeframe for correction. Thus the most complex will likely take the longest, but the timeframe helps to set both limits to the negative activities and goals for the incorporation of the positive corrections. Only by taking action does the evaluation process of quality assessment reach the goal of quality assurance.

The cultivation of evaluation is a critical component of a professional dental hygienist's skills. Evaluation programs are designed to guarantee excellence in dental hygiene care. They enable the dental hygiene professional to be accountable to society for the quality of service provided. It also identifies those actions that the hygienist successfully performed that impacted on the client's health status. Evaluation programs help to define the dental hygiene process and scope of dental hygiene practice uniquely performed by the dental hygienist.

REFERENCES

American Dental Hygienists' Association. (1985). *Standards of applied dental hygiene practice.* Chicago, IL: American Dental Hygienists' Association.

Burt, B., & Eklund, S. (1992). *Dentistry, dental practice and the community,* Philadelphia: W.B. Saunders Company.

Donabedian, A. (1982). *The criteria and standards of quality, Vol. 2, Exploration in quality assessment and monitoring.* Ann Arbor, MI: Health Administration Press.

Gaston, M.A. (1994, May). Proposed draft code of ethics for dental hygiene. *Access, 8,* 3–10.

Ingersoll, B. (1982). *Behavioral aspects in dentistry.* New York: Appleton-Century-Crofts.

Morris, A.L., Bentley, J.M., Vito, A.A., & Bomba, M.R. (1988). Assessment of private dental practice: Report of a study. *Journal of the American Dental Association, 117*, 153–162.

Schoen, M.H., Freed, J., Gershen, J.A.Q., & Marcus, M. (1989). Appendix: Guidelines for criteria and standards of acceptable quality general dental practice (special emphasis on group practice). *Journal of Dental Education, 53*, 662–669.

Exercise 7.1   Types of Evaluation

Categorize the following into the type of evaluation—structural, (S), process (P), or outcome (O)—by placing the correct letter on the line provided. Some statements may fit into more than one category.

_____ 1. Evaluation of instruments indicates all periodontal scalers are dull.

_____ 2. Client returns five days following a full mouth ultrasonic scaling with a periodontal abscess.

_____ 3. Hygienist is frequently "running late" by 10 or 15 minutes.

_____ 4. Clients are waiting four to six weeks for a recall appointment with the hygienist.

_____ 5. Client did not comply with the recommended fluoride regimen.

_____ 6. Hygienist must lose a day's salary in order to take a continuing education course.

_____ 7. The most recent entry in a client's chart is as follows:

_____   1/18/94 Px, FlTx EJG

_____ 8. Assessment of a client at the four-month recall reveals a high plaque and bleeding score.

_____ 9. Client's chart indicates that the size and location of a keratinized lesion in the buccal vestibule was noted by the previous hygienist. No other notation is made.

_____ 10. Hygienist uses poor infection control technique with daylight loader on automatic film processor.

Exercise 7.2   Managing an Evaluation

For each of the situations listed in Exercise 7.1 identify what appears to be the main problem. When that is identified, what questions need to be asked to determine what course(s) of action needs to be taken to correct the problem.

> Sample: Evaluation of instruments indicates all periodontal scalers are dull.
>
> Problem: Dull scalers reduce efficiency.
>
> Questions: Who is responsible for the task? Why are the scalers not being sharpened? Is it a lack of knowledge, time, or attitude? Who should be responsible?

Once some of these initial questions are asked, how will the problem be corrected? Does each clinician know how to sharpen instruments properly? Are there sufficient sharpening stones or other devices available? Are sterile stones available during appointments? Is time allotted to evaluate instruments? What methods are used to evaluate sharpness? Are all instruments in the practice available for "community" use or are some personal property of each clinician?

Should a formal procedure be instituted in which instruments are evaluated periodically and a replacement schedule instituted? Continue with the situations listed in Exercise 7.1, using the format of problem identification and a list of possible questions.

APPENDIX A: CASE STUDIES

INTRODUCTION

The cases that follow are designed to enable the reader to work through the dental hygiene care process. Assessment information will lead the reader through the process of decision making, formulating diagnostic statements, selecting dental hygiene interventions, writing expected outcomes of treatment, and care planning. At the conclusion of each case you are given the opportunity to develop a sample appointment plan based on the individualized client's plan of care.

There are four cases in total. Each case begins with a narrative statement providing some subjective data about the client. Assessment findings are listed and questions will guide you through to diagnostic decision making. Answers can be found in the text of the case and will provide additional information when necessary. The format of the cases vary, although the context is the same. Spaces are provided for your answers.

FINAL CASE 1   MR. GEORGE FLOWERS

Narrative

George Flowers is a 38-year-old man who has not been to the dentist in over five years. He completes the medical history form in the waiting room and is seated for the initial assessment appointment.

Assessment Findings (Appointment #1)

MEDICAL HISTORY

Client indicates the presence of mitral valve prolapse and hypertension. Client is taking Diazide to control hypertension.

Before continuing with the assessment what questions should be asked?

_____

_____

_____

_____

_____

Answer: Have you ever taken antibiotic premedication prior to dental procedures before? Are you aware that you are at risk for bacterial endocarditis, which can be life threatening? Is your blood pressure under control? When was the last time you had a physical examination?

Upon further questioning the client indicates that he has never been premedicated prior to dental treatment and is unaware of the dangers involved. The client is also a little apprehensive about taking an antibiotic for prevention.

At this point could a dental hygiene diagnosis be made? _____

If yes, write a dental hygiene diagnostic statement based on the above assessment findings.

_____

_____

_____

_____

Yes, The dental hygiene diagnostic statement related to the above assessment finding would be:

Anxiety related to need for antibiotic premedication

Fill in the following information:

Goal Statements	Dental Hygiene Interventions	Expected Outcomes

Answer:

Goal Statement	Dental Hygiene Interventions	Expected Outcomes
Relieve anxiety related to antibiotic premedication Increase client's awareness concerning risks involved with infective endocarditis	1. Educate on possible risks involved with infective endocarditis 2. Consult with dentist for antibiotic premedication prescription	1. Client will take antibiotic premedication prior to dental hygiene appointment

(continues)

3. Call client prior to next
   dental hygiene appointment
   to remind him of
   premedication

4. Contact client's physician
   to alert him of the need for
   premedication for some
   dental procedures

At this point should client continue to be treated or reappointed?

_____

Could any other assessment procedures be performed? _____
If yes, which ones:

_____

_____

_____

_____

Answer:
Extra oral examination
Oral hygiene evaluation
Radiographic survey

EXTRA ORAL EXAMINATION
WNL

ORAL HYGIENE EVALUATION
Plaque index revealed that plaque was present on 80% of all interproximal surfaces and 90% of all lingual surfaces.

What additional questions should be asked?

_____

_____

_____

_____

_____

Answer:
What is your home care regimen?
What type of dental products do you use?

Further questioning reveals that Mr. Flowers brushes at least once daily in the AM. He does not floss because the contacts are too tight. He does not use any other type of dental product besides toothpaste.

RADIOGRAPHIC SURVEY

Multiple areas of vertical bone loss; no radiographic evidence of caries

The client is then reappointed and given a prescription for antibiotic premedication with instructions for use prior to the next dental hygiene appointment

Assessment Findings (Appointment #2):

The client informs the dental hygienist that he has taken the prescribed antibiotic premedication. This information must be recorded in the client's chart.

DENTAL EXAM

No clinical evidence of dental caries or decalcification. Several small restorations are found on the occlusal surfaces of teeth #2, #3, #14, #15, #19, #30.

PERIODONTAL EXAM

Significant findings related to the periodontal exam are listed below.

Pocket Depth: Pocket depth ranges from 4 mm to 5 mm in all posterior sextants.

Attachment Loss: Enlargement of the interdental papilla reveals that true attachment loss ranges from 3 mm to 4 mm in all posterior sextants.

Bleeding on Probing: Interproximal bleeding on probing is present in all posterior sextants.

Suppuration: No evidence of suppuration

Mobility: No evidence of mobility

Furcation Involvement: No evidence of furcation involvement

GINGIVAL EXAM

Clinical findings reveal localized inflammation of the posterior interproximal papilla. All other areas remain WNL.

DEPOSIT CLASSIFICATION

Supragingival Calculus: Light accumulation found on the lingual surfaces of the mandibular anterior teeth.

Subgingival Calculus: Moderate interproximal calculus found on the interproximal surfaces of all posterior teeth.

Plaque and Stain: Minimal stain and moderate interproximal plaque accumulation present.

DIAGNOSTIC TESTS

**DNA analysis of plaque sample revealed high levels of periodontal pathogens.

Based on these assessment findings write two dental hygiene diagnostic statements that would be relevant:

_____

_____

_____

_____

_____

_____

_____

_____

Answer: Considering the assessment findings, the following are sample dental hygiene diagnostic statements. You may have worded them differently but check for content.

1. Bleeding on probing related to subgingival deposits and ineffective interproximal plaque control
2. Potential for reduced bone level related to high levels of periodontal pathogens

Fill in the following information for Diagnostic Statement #1:

Goal Statements	Dental Hygiene Interventions	Expected Outcomes

Answer: Diagnostic Statement #1

Goal Statements	Dental Hygiene Interventions	Expected Outcomes
Elimination of interproximal bleeding	1. Evaluate client's tooth-brushing technique and modify accordingly 2. Educate client on the importance of inter-proximal plaque control 3. Demonstrate use of waxed dental floss 4. Recommend the use of an antimicrobial mouthrinse to be used twice daily (AM and PM) as part of home care regimen 5. Scale deposits with the use of hand and ultra-sonic instruments 6. Take plaque index	1. Client will demonstrate revised or new technique and incorporate its use in daily home care practices 2. Client will use waxed dental floss once daily for two weeks 3. Client will rinse with an antimicrobial mouth rinse twice daily as part of home regimen for two weeks 4. Evaluate deposit removal with subgingival explorer 5. Client will reduce plaque score by 50%

Now complete the following chart for Diagnostic Statement #2:

Goal Statements	Dental Hygiene Interventions	Expected Outcomes

Answer: Diagnostic Statement #2

Goal Statements	Dental Hygiene Interventions	Expected Outcomes
Maintain present bone level	1. Monitor changes in the bone level via radiographs and probing depth measurements 2. If significant changes in bone level occurs provide more aggressive therapy, i.e., subgingival irrigation, extensive subgingival debridement. Consult DDS for use of systemic antibiotics, etc. 3. Monitor client's home care practices via daily diary cards, frequent recall 4. Assess and monitor levels of periodontal pathogens via plaque sampling and DNA probing	1. Bone level will be maintained at its present level for the next three months 2. Client will perform home care regimen 2x daily and record in diary 3. Client will return for maintenance therapy in three months 4. Pathogen levels will remain low by evidence of DNA probe diagnostic test at three months

Now review the dental hygiene interventions listed previously and complete the appointment plan.

APPOINTMENT PLAN

_____

_____

_____

_____

_____

_____

_____

_____

_____

_____

_____

_____

_____

_____

_____

_____

_____

_____

_____

_____

_____

_____

_____

_____

Answer: The following is a sample appointment plan for the dental hygiene interventions listed in the care plan. Remember that the appointment plan consists only of interventions, not assessment procedures.

APPOINTMENT PLAN

Appointment #1 (1 hour)

1. Validate client's premedication
2. Evaluate client's toothbrushing technique and modify if necessary
3. Educate the client on the importance of interproximal plaque control
4. Demonstrate use of waxed dental floss
5. Recommend the use of an antimicrobial mouthrinse to be used twice daily following home care regimen
6. Scale deposits found in the mandibular and maxillary right quadrants

Appointment #2 (1 1/2 hour / 2 weeks)

1. Validate client's premedication
2. Review client's home care practices
3. Scale remaining areas mandibular left and maxillary right quadrants
4. Selectively polish
5. Fluoride treatment
6. Reappoint for 3 months

Appointment #3 (1 hour / 3 months)

1. Evaluate client's home care practices with indices
2. Reassess periodontal condition via clinical and microbial evaluation
3. Scale any deposits that have accumulated
4. Make decision concerning maintenance options: i.e., continue, add aggressive therapies, refer

FINAL CASE 2   LYNN WILKINSON

Narrative

Lynn Wilkinson is 26 years old and in her sixth month of her first pregnancy. After she is seated, she indicates she is here because her gums have been very sore and for the last week or so have bled a lot when she brushed. She says she hasn't brushed too well in the last several days due to the discomfort. She says she is concerned because she knows "that pregnancy contributes to tooth loss because all the calcium goes to the baby," but she hopes that won't happen to her. Her last dental visit was two years ago for a cleaning just before her wedding. She states that she really thinks she has "good teeth" because she has very few fillings and hasn't needed any for a long time.

Assessment Findings (Appointment #1)

The client's medical history is good. She is having an uneventful pregnancy. Her chart indicates that she had her teeth scaled twenty-two months previously. It was noted then that the hygienist gave oral hygiene instruction. Her radiographs from the previous visit indicates only three molars with restorations, two occlusal amalgams, and MOD on tooth 19. All seem radiographically to be sound with no marginal overhangs on #19. The extra oral exam indicates all within normal limits. Her intra oral examination, however, indicates edematous papillae in about 50% of the mouth, bleeding on probing throughout, and a high plaque score. Light subgingival calculus is present. Probe depths are greater than those recorded previously, but this appears to be a result of the pseudo-pockets due to edematous tissue.

Before continuing, since this case constitutes an "emergency," what considerations or actions would you include at this point?

_____

_____

_____

_____

_____

_____

_____

_____

_____

Answer: 1) Since the main concern of this visit is to alleviate the symptoms and return the client to proper function, the emphasis must be on clinical interventions. Home care instructions should focus on immediate support of clinical actions with more long-term behavioral interventions reserved for a future appointment. 2) Decision needed on whether radiographs are necessary at this point. Given the client's dental history, they may not be necessary; however, in this trimester four bitewings taken with all appropriate safety precautions would be acceptable. Bone level comparisons should be made to assist in the diagnosis. This decision can also be postponed to the next visit following reassessment.

Write two dental hygiene diagnoses for this client.

1. _____

_____

_____

_____

_____

2. _____

_____

_____

_____

_____

Answer:

   1. Gingivitis related to the hormonal effects of pregnancy and inadequate home care

   2. Potential for compromised oral health related to health beliefs

Write a goal statement for this case:

_____

_____

_____

Answer:

    Eliminate contributory causes of inflammation through clinical and behavioral interventions and educate the client on the role of plaque control and its implications for oral health. Increase the client's overall oral health knowledge to effect a change in beliefs.

Would you attempt to institute all the goals at the first appointment? _____

Answer: No. Due to the emergency situation, the client needs to have immediate concerns solved before any extensive change can take place. However, as symptoms exacerbate, the timing will be ideal to institute behavior change that may be long term. The first sentence of the goal paragraph directs the early care in this sample.

Using the format below fill in the following information.

Goal Statement	Dental Hygiene Interventions	Expected Outcomes

Answer:

Goal Statement	Dental Hygiene Interventions	Expected Outcomes
Eliminate contributory causes of inflammatory response	1. Periodontal debridement 2. Irrigate	1. Bleeding on probing will be reduced in 75 percent of sites
Discuss plaque control measures	1. Demonstrate techniques 2. Relate plaque to current problem	1. Client will brush twice daily and floss daily

At the follow-up visit in one week, Lynn shows a healthy response to the interventions. She claims she is brushing as you showed her and flossing, although that is still giving her some difficulty. At this point what diagnostic statement can be made?

Answer: Your diagnostic statement should look similar to the following—

Knowledge and skill deficit related to plaque control program.

Fill in the following table based on your new diagnostic statement:

Goal Statement	Dental Hygiene Interventions	Expected Outcomes

Answer:

Goal Statement	Dental Hygiene Interventions	Expected Outcomes
	1. Reassess tissue response 2. Take Plaque Index 3. Correct problems	
Increase overall knowledge of oral health to well-being	1. Relate relationship of oral symptoms to general health	1. Identify oral health parameters
Acknowledge role as mother and impact on child's oral health	2. Discuss infant oral health	2. Describe oral health for baby

If this client had not responded well to therapy, what would you have done?

Answer:

If the client was still showing evidence of inflammation following a thorough scaling, consultation with the dentist and/or the client's obstetrician would be necessary.

Design a plan that includes the services performed at the first and second appoint-ments. Decide on a recall maintenance appointment schedule and its plan.

APPOINTMENT PLAN

_____

_____

_____

_____

_____

_____

_____

_____

_____

_____

_____

_____

_____

Answer:

APPOINTMENT PLAN

Appointment #1 (1 Hour)

Following initial assessment and diagnosis:

1. Complete periodontal debridement
2. Irrigate
3. Initiate oral hygiene instruction, Bass technique

Appointment #2 (45 minutes   1 week later)

1. Reassess; evaluate tissue response to therapy
2. Debride any areas not thoroughly responding to therapy
3. Irrigate
4. Continue behavioral interventions to assist client to maintain habit following emergency motivation. Ascertain client goals, use contract or daily charting to help monitor implementation of new habit. Provide reading matter for the oral care of infants and children
5. If tissue has responded well reappoint in two months before birth
6. If there are still unresolved sites, reappoint in one to two weeks for 15 to 30 minutes

Appointment #3 (2 month maintenance visit)

1. Reassess
2. Include education, answer questions on oral hygiene care of infants

FINAL CASE 3   LEROY MILLER

Narrative

Leroy Miller is seventy years old. He indicates that he has "bad breath" and a dry mouth and has been using "mints to alleviate the problem." He indicates that he is having difficulty brushing because his arthritis is making it difficult to grasp the toothbrush. He proudly indicates that he still has all of his teeth and has always taken very good care of his mouth, receiving regular dental care annually. He has been coming to this dental office for twenty years but this is the first time you will be treating him.

Assessment Findings (Appointment #1)

The client's medical history indicates that he is taking 50 mg of Diazide once a day to control hypertension. His current blood pressure reading is 123/82. He has thirty-two teeth, several with gold onlays or inlays, and two amalgams that are blackened in appearance. There is toothbrush abrasion on the buccal surfaces of all posterior teeth, particularly on teeth #11, #12, #13, #20, and #21. There is slight supragingival calculus on crowded mandibular posterior teeth and attrition. There is generalized gingival recession of 1 to 2 mm. Pocket depth readings are <3 mm on the anterior teeth and increasing pocket depth of 4 mm on the posterior teeth. There is plaque accumulation on the lingual surfaces of maxillary and mandibular posterior teeth. During the assessment you not the dry mucosa and slightly fissured tongue.

List the problems evident in the client that you would consider to be part of the dental diagnosis.

_____

_____

_____

Answer: Xerostomia, toothbrush abrasion, oxidized amalgam, plaque accumulation, halitosis

What additional clarifications would be necessary for each of the problems listed before any decisions can be made?

Xerostomia _____

_____

_____

Toothbrush abrasion _____

_____

_____

Plaque accumulation _____

_____

_____

Halitosis _____

_____

_____

Oxidized amalgams _____

_____

_____

Dental sensitivity _____

_____

_____

Answers:

Xerostomia: Aging is a factor, however Diazide may also be a contributing factor. Therefore, question how long the drug has been taken; was the dry mouth evident before the drug was prescribed? When was his last doctor's visit? Did he discuss this with him? What type of "mints" is he using? Is he doing anything else to alleviate the symptoms?

Toothbrush abrasion: Was the abrasion previously noted on the chart? If so, is the client aware and has the technique been altered? Is there any sensitivity? Does the appearance disturb the client? Has anyone discussed restorations with him?

Plaque accumulation: Evaluate current technique. Can moderations be made to a standard brush? Would a mechanical toothbrush be more effective? Has a floss holder been recommended?

Halitosis: The plaque accumulation on teeth may be contributing to the problem. Is client brushing tongue as well as teeth? Since there may be a medical cause, re-evaluation will be necessary following resolution of the plaque accumulation problem.

Oxidized amalgam: The problem is caused by the galvanic reaction of the metals. No additional information is necessary.

Dental sensitivity: The exposed root surfaces and/or CEJ are causing sensitivity.

CLIENT RESPONSES

Xerostomia: Mr. Miller has been taking the drug for one year. He thinks maybe that was when he noted the dryness starting. He is using a variety of mints, but mostly sugarless ones. He needs to have water at his bedside, because the dryness in his mouth wakes him and he is uncomfortable. Explain that you can help alleviate some of the symptoms, however he should discuss the condition with his physician.

Toothbrush abrasion: The abrasion was previously noted on the chart. Mr. Miller is aware of it. Previously he used a hard natural bristle toothbrush because that was what was recommended many years ago. He currently uses a soft bristle toothbrush and claims to brush the way he was taught. He does not like the way #11 looks when he smiles, but doesn't want the tooth to be drilled for a restoration. When questioned about sensitivity, the client claims some sensitivity to cold.

Plaque accumulation: Mr. Miller's brushing technique is quite good within the limitations that his arthritis is imposing. Turning his hand into the lingual regions is limiting his access. He is very motivated. Flossing has become very difficult.

Halitosis: Plaque and food particles left on teeth and tongue may be the sole factor. Mr. Miller said no one ever told him about brushing his tongue.

Oxidized amalgams: Show client the amalgams. Indicate the cause and explain the polishing procedure that will hopefully restore their appearance and prolong function.

Dental sensitivity: Mr. Miller states that cold drinks or ice cream sometimes cause a sensitivity.

Dental Hygiene Diagnosis

Write a diagnostic statement(s) for each of the problems identified.

1. _____

_____

_____

_____

_____

2. _____

_____

_____

_____

3. _____

_____

_____

_____

4. _____

_____

_____

_____

_____

5. _____

_____

_____

_____

_____

6. _____

_____

_____

_____

_____

Answer:

1. A. Decreased salivary flow related to aging and hypertensive medication
   B. Potential for decay related to xerostomia and gingival recession
2. Toothbrush abrasion related to incorrect technique
3. Oxidized amalgam related to galvanic reaction of different metals used in restorations
4. Plaque accumulation related to reduced dexterity in plaque control
5. Halitosis related to knowledge deficit and reduced dexterity
6. Dental sensitivity related to exposed root surfaces

For each of the diagnostic statements fill in the following information.

Diagnostic Statement #1

Goal Statement	Dental Hygiene Interventions	Expected Outcomes

Answer:

Goal Statement	Dental Hygiene Interventions	Expected Outcomes
Increase client's comfort through use of artificial saliva	1. Educate on use of artificial saliva	1. Client will use artificial saliva
Reduce potential for decay	1. Educate regarding use of fluoride	2. Client will use OTC fluoride rinse daily

Diagnostic Statement #2

Goal Statement	Dental Hygiene Interventions	Expected Outcomes

Answer:

Goal Statement	Dental Hygiene Interventions	Expected Outcomes
Educate client regarding bonded type restoration	1. Refer client to dentist	1. Client will decide following consult with DDS

Diagnostic Statement #3

Goal Statement	Dental Hygiene Interventions	Expected Outcomes

Answer:

Goal Statement	Dental Hygiene Interventions	Expected Outcomes
Reduce/eliminate oxidation	1. Polish amalgams	1. Appearance/ life of restoration will be prolonged

Diagnostic Statement #4

Goal Statement	Dental Hygiene Interventions	Expected Outcomes

Answer:

Goal Statement	Dental Hygiene Interventions	Expected Outcomes
Reduce plaque accumulation by using oral physiotherapy aids	1. Modify toothbrush using bike handle grip and angling head of brush 2. Demonstrate floss holder	1. Client will have improved plaque score

Diagnostic Statement #5

Goal Statement	Dental Hygiene Interventions	Expected Outcomes

Answer:

Goal Statement	Dental Hygiene Interventions	Expected Outcomes
Increase client's knowledge regarding plaque reduction on tongue	1. Demonstrate technique of brushing tongue daily	1. Client will clean tongue

Diagnostic Statement #6

Goal Statement	Dental Hygiene Interventions	Expected Outcomes

Answer:

Goal Statement	Dental Hygiene Interventions	Expected Outcomes
Reduce dental sensitivity	1. Educate client regarding cause and methods to reduce sensitivity	1. Client will use desensitizing toothpaste for one month
	2. Provide in-office desensitizing treatment	In-office desensitizing treatment will provide temporary relief of sensitivity

How many appointments would need to be scheduled with Mr. Miller? What maintenance interval should be scheduled?

APPOINTMENT PLAN

_____

_____

_____

_____

_____

_____

Answer:

Assuming the normal appointment time is forty-five minutes to an hour, this client would most likely have his dental hygiene therapy completed in one appointment. It would be advisable to see Mr. Miller in one month to evaluate the effects of the saliva substitutes and plaque control. If the halitosis continues following improved plaque control, the client should be advised to seek medical care to rule out any physiological causes.

FINAL CASE 4 BLAIR McKLEMENT

Narrative

Blair McKlement is a 16-year-old high school student. She has been a client of the practice for the past 10 years and her last maintenance appointment was 2 years ago.

Assessment Findings

MEDICAL HISTORY
WNL

EXTRA-ORAL EXAM
WNL, Physical appearance underweight

INTRA-ORAL EXAM
Palatal petecchia

What additional questions may be asked at this point?

_____

_____

_____

_____

_____

_____

_____

_____

Answer:

1. Are you trying to lose weight?
2. Does your palate(roof of your mouth) hurt?
3. Have you eaten anything sharp like potato chips?

DENTAL EXAM

Lingual erosion of maxillary anterior teeth

Deep pits and fissures on all occlusal surfaces of the posterior teeth

What additional probing questions may be asked at this point?

_____

_____

_____

_____

_____

_____

_____

_____

Answers:

Some probing questions based on your dental exam might be:

1. Do you vomit frequently?
2. Do you eat or suck on a lot of citrus fruits such as lemons, or grapefruits?
3. What constitutes your diet?

Following this question period Blair states that she does vomit frequently.

What could be possible causes of frequent vomiting?

_____

_____

_____

_____

_____

_____

_____

_____

_____

_____

Answers:

Some suggested answers would include:

1. pregnancy
2. bulimia
3. gastrointestinal disturbance

Further questioning revealed that Blair is extremely self-conscious about her weight and admits she occasionally induces vomiting after eating to get rid of the food.

Based on the above assessment findings what nutritional disorder may be present? and why?

_____

_____

_____

_____

_____

_____

_____

_____

_____

_____

Answer: According to the assessment findings, Blair most likely has the nutritional eating disorder bulimia. The oral manifestations of bulimia are palatal petecchia from objects used to induce vomiting and erosion of lingual surfaces of the maxillary anteriors due to frequent regurgitation. Bulimia affects females more than males and is common among high school and college age women who are self-conscious about their appearance.

At this point could any dental hygiene diagnosis be made? _____

If yes, write the dental diagnostic statements associated with the above assessment findings.

_____

_____

_____

_____

_____

_____

_____

Answer: Yes, the dental hygiene diagnostic statements related to the above assessment findings would be:

1. Erosion of anterior teeth related to nutritional eating disorder
2. Potential for occlusal decay related to deep occlusal pits and fissures

Fill in the following information for Diagnostic Statement #1

Goal Statement	Dental Hygiene Interventions	Expected Outcomes

Answer:

Goal Statement	Dental Hygiene Interventions	Expected Outcomes
Eliminate continued erosion of maxillary anterior teeth	1. Educate client on importance of good nutrition for overall health as well as dental health	1. Client will be able to identify nutritional disturbances in general and oral health
	2. Counsel client on good nutritional habits	2. Client will be able to choose foods that are nutritionally sound
	3. Advise and assist client to seek counseling	3. Client will improve nutritional habits
	4. Provide support for body image change	4. Client will seek counseling

Fill in the following information for Diagnostic Statement #2

Goal Statement	Dental Hygiene Interventions	Expected Outcomes

Answer:

Goal Statement	Dental Hygiene Interventions	Expected Outcomes
Decrease risk for occlusal decay	1. Educate client on risk of occlusal decay and the decay process	1. Client will recognize risk of occlusal decay by understanding the decay process
	2. Sealant application for all molar teeth	2. All molar teeth will be appropriately sealed by using light cured sealant

PERIODONTAL EXAM
WNL

GINGIVAL EXAM
WNL

ORAL HYGIENE EVALUATION
Plaque Index indicated that plaque is present on 7 percent of all tooth surfaces.
    What additional questions should be asked?

_____

_____

_____

_____

Answer:
Tell me when you usually brush your teeth.
    Blair states that she usually brushes in the AM and PM but was in a hurry this morning and did not get a chance to brush her teeth.
    What would you do, ask Blair to brush her teeth now or continue to perform your assessment?

_____

_____

_____

_____

Answer: Ask Blair to brush her teeth so you can evaluate her brushing technique.

Blair's brushing technique is adequate. She seems to remove most of the accumulated plaque.

Complete the following appointment plan based on your diagnostic statements and assessment findings.

APPOINTMENT PLAN

_____

_____

_____

_____

_____

_____

_____

_____

_____

_____

_____

_____

_____

_____

_____

Answer:

The following Appointment Plan is based on the assessment findings and diagnostic statements developed in this case.

APPOINTMENT PLAN

Appointment #1 (one hour)

1. Educate client on risk of occlusal decay and the decay process
2. Discuss with client the need for sealants on the molar teeth
3. Educate client on importance of good nutrition for overall health as well as dental health
4. Advise client to seek counseling for nutritional eating disorder
5. Deplaque all teeth

Appointment #2 (forty-five minutes)

1. Provide support for body image change
2. Assess progress of counseling
3. Apply sealant to all teeth
4. Discuss daily use of home fluoride therapy

Reappoint for maintenance six months
Follow-up call one month to discuss progress in counseling

APPENDIX B: ANSWERS TO EXERCISES

Exercise 1.3 (p. 18)

1. I
2. I
3. I
4. I
5. I
6. I/D
7. I
8. IT
9. D
10. IT
11. I
12. IT
13. I

Exercise 1.4 (p 19)

1. C
2. A
3. D
4. E
5. B

Exercise 2.1 (p. 44)

1. O
2. O
3. S
4. S
5. O
6. S
7. O
8. O
9. S
10. O
11. H
12. C
13. H
14. C
15. C
16. H
17. H
18. H
19. C
20. C

Exercise 2.2 (p. 45)

2
1
3
5
4

Exercise 2.3 (p. 45)

Finding	Risk Factor	Medical Clearance or Premedication	Continue Comprehensive Charting
Example: Client reports mitral valve prolapse	Subacute bacterial endocarditis	Yes	No
Diabetes	Poor healing	Yes	Yes
Hypotension	Syncope	No	Yes
Pregnancy	Hormonal exaggeration of periodontal condition	No	Yes

Exercise 3.1 (p. 64)

1. E
2. C
3. A
4. B
5. D

Exercise 3.2 (p. 64)

A. Increased plaque accumulation related to flossing knowledge deficit
B. Tooth sensitivity related to presence of toothbrush abrasion (or exposed dentin)
C. Increased oral deposits related to limited dexterity

Exercise 3.3 (p. 65)

1. **Diagnostic Statement:**

   Altered alveolar bone level related to active periodontal condition.

   Assessment Findings:

   - Radiographic evidence of horizontal and vertical bone loss
   - Bleeding upon probing
   - Suppuration
   - Probing depths greater than 4 mm
   - DNA probe evidence of high levels of periodontal pathogens

2. **Diagnostic Statement:**

Chronic lymphadenopathy related to partial third molar eruption

Assessment Findings:

- Extra oral finding of palpable nodes right side
- Intra oral finding of partial eruption of mandibular right third molar
- Client's subjective statement of pain on right side
- Gingival assessment of inflamed operculum
- Debris accumulation under operculum

3. **Diagnostic Statement:**

Maxillary incisal decay related to improper bottle feeding

Assessment Findings:

- Intra oral finding of maxillary incisal decay
- Nutritional questioning of parent revels that the child is constantly using a bottle with various liquids; juice, milk, or water
- Client habits include thumb sucking and sleeping with a bottle usually filled with milk
- Oral hygiene is limited to occasional toothbrushing

Exercise 4.1 (p. 87)

1. Primary, specific protection
2. Primary, specific protection
3. Tertiary, disability limitation
4. Tertiary, disability limitation
5. Tertiary, disability limitation
6. Primary, health promotion
7. Secondary, early diagnosis and treatment
8. Secondary, early diagnosis and treatment

Exercise 4.2 (p. 87)

Description	Defining Characteristic	Risk Factor
Sulcular bleeding	X	
Poor oral hygiene		X
Excessive exposure to sun for fair-skinned individual		X
Use of juice bottle at baby's bedtime		X
High sucrose intake		X
Decay of maxillary central incisors of a three-year-old	X	
Elevated diastolic blood pressure reading	X	
Mottled enamel	X	

Exercise 4.3 (p. 88)

1. Here is a sample list with pros and cons identified. Your list may differ to some degree, which is expected.

    Cost – con

    Speech while under treatment – con

    Appearance – pro and con

    Discomfort of treatment – con

    Scheduling appointments – pro or con

    Length of time – pro or con

    Pain of headaches reduced – pro

    Potential future oral problems – pro

    Self-esteem – pro

    Smile quality – pro

    Opinion of others – pro and/or con

2. Pros and Cons. Once again, your opinion of an attribute may differ from the one supplied—that doesn't mean yours is incorrect. However, you should think about the attribute, if it does differ, to open your mind to the contrary opinion.

3. Weights. The ones determined "serious" should be reviewed. With a client at this point, all that can be done is to be satisfied that as a professional you

have helped identify important issues and pointed the client in a direction that is of value. But, it is the client's decision. By enabling the client to make the decision and feel part of the decision-making process, clients will be more likely to be satisfied and comply with recommendations.

Exercise 5.1 (p. 107)

__S__   __P__   __CD__

1. Inflammation will be eliminated by the removal of denture for

   __CR__

   6 to 8 hours daily.

   _____S_____   ____P____

2. Potential for infection of third molar area will be reduced by

   __CR__   __CD__

   the daily use of irrigation

Exercise 5.2 (p. 107)

1. Observation — 2 weeks
2. Apply plaque score —1 week and at intervals thereafter
3. Client keeps five-day diet diary
4. Keep daily chart for 1 month to establish habit
5. Compare probe readings to baseline

Exercise 5.3 (p. 107)

Limit further damage of mucosal tissue and cease the use of smokeless tobacco

List the dental hygiene interventions that would be appropriate:

1. Evaluate client's current knowledge
2. Demonstrate adverse effects in mouth
3. Set goal for reduction and elimination of smokeless tobacco use
4. Explore safe alternatives
5. Establish a plan to monitor behavioral change
6. Refer for oral pathology consultation

Establish an appointment plan:

Visit 1: Provide education regarding smokeless tobacco
           Set goal and outcomes with client
           Teach oral cancer self-examination

Visit 2: Review and evaluate progress to goal
           Establish appropriate oral cancer re-evaluation

Exercise 6.1 (p. 123)

1. semicritical
2. noncritical
3. noncritical
4. noncritical
5. semicritical
6. critical
7. noncritical
8. semicritical
9. noncritical
10. critical

Exercise 6.2 (p. 123)

The problem is based in the area of motivation. There are many ways to increase a client's motivational level. You only had to identify three. Here are a few possible answers.

Change behavior environments

Add reminders

Obtain written commitment

Positive reinforcement

Reward program

Identify consequences

Exercise 7.1 (p. 139)

1. process and/or structure
2. process
3. structure
4. structure
5. outcome
6. structure
7. process/structure
8. outcome
9. process
10. process

Exercise 7.2 (p. 140)

2. Problem: The assumption is that "gross scaling" does not thoroughly remove the deposit contributing to a partial healing of the cervical gingiva with disease remaining active at the base of the pocket.

   Question: What protocol change would reduce the probability of this occurring again? Is the appointment schedule time sufficient to provide comprehensive care? Does the hygienist have adequate technical skill and knowledge of the disease process to implement quality care? If yes, what methods will be employed to correct this inadequacy?

3. Problem possibilities: 1. Appointment time is insufficient to permit time for the hygienist to perform the necessary functions and services. 2. Hygienist is inefficient (i.e., too talkative or disorganized).

   Questions: Should appointment time be increased or should hygienist plan to provide treatment in more than one appointment? Should fees be adjusted to complement an increase in services? What specific changes need too be implemented to increase efficiency? Are the changes with the personnel or procedures? (i.e., Can the roving assistant process the radiographs for the hygienist?)

4. Problem: Personnel is not available to accommodate potential clients.

   Questions: Should the current hygienist(s) work additional hours or days? Should additional personnel be hired?

5. Problem: The expected outcome did not meet the actual outcome. Since the client did not comply, the assumption in this case would be that the client's goals need to be evaluated. See checklist in Table 7.3 to assess the questions that may be asked.

6. Problem: The structure does not support continuing education.

   Questions: Is this continuing education course necessary to improve client care? What issues need to be negotiated with the employer so that the goal of participating in courses by the hygienist does not result in lost pay?

7. Problem: Chart entry is inadequate to support a legal challenge. It does not communicate to other team members at subsequent appointments what has transpired.

   Questions: Does the structure of record keeping discourage more complete recording of client data? Does the hygienist have sufficient knowledge of risk management requirements? Is the hygienist delivering quality care?

8. Problem: Actual outcome did not meet expected outcome. In this case a number of causes might be contributing. It would be necessary to review the entire care plan using checklists in Tables, 7.2, 7.3, 7.4, and 7.5.

9. Problem: The chart entry is incomplete in terms of description of the lesion and does not indicate if the client was informed, if a referral was made, or what follow-up was planned. Similar to #7 above; the legal as well as ethical issues are important to address.

10. Problem: The hygienist is using poor technique.

    Questions: Is the cause a lack of knowledge? Is the equipment, number of gloves provided or other cause in the structure prohibiting adequate technique?

INDEX